Blood Picture

Richard H. Nollan

Blood Picture

L. W. Diggs, Sickle Cell Anemia, and the South's First Blood Bank

The University of Tennessee Press
Knoxville

All images courtesy of the Health Science Historical Collections, Library and Bio-communications Center, University of Tennessee Health Science Center, Memphis.

Library of Congress Cataloging-in-Publication Data
Names: Nollan, Richard.
Title: Blood picture : L.W. Diggs, sickle cell anemia, and the South's first blood bank / Richard H. Nollan.
Description: Knoxville : The University of Tennessee Press, [2016] | Includes bibliographical references and index.
Identifiers: LCCN 2015039612 | ISBN 9781621902218 (hardcover : alk. paper)
Subjects: LCSH: Diggs, L. W. (Lemuel W.), 1900-1995. | St. Jude Children's Research Hospital. | Physicians—United States—Biography. | Sickle cell anemia—Treatment. | Blood banks—Tennessee.
Classification: LCC R154.D5525 N65 2016 | DDC 610.92—dc23
LC record available at http://lccn.loc.gov/2015039612

Lay me on an anvil, O God."
Beat me and hammer me into a crowbar.
Let me pry loose old walls.
Let me lift and loosen old foundations.

Lay me on an anvil, O God.
Beat me and hammer me into a steel spike.
Drive me into the girders that hold a skyscraper together.
Take red-hot rivets and fasten me into the central girders.
Let me be the great nail holding a skyscraper through blue
    nights into white stars.

—Carl Sandburg, "Prayers of Steel," *Cornhuskers*, 1918

A clipping of this poem appeared to have been entered into a commonplace
book by Diggs's fiancée, Beatrice Mosher, with the comment, "Here is a poem
I found that seemed to crystallize your attitude toward going there. It is Carl
Sandburg's maybe you've heard it." The comment was probably written on the
occasion of their move to Memphis. The commonplace book can be found
in: 1779 Diggs, L. W. 1999.

Contents

Illustrations

Acknowledgments

The threads of sickle cell anemia, blood transfusion, and laboratory medicine are bound up in the figure of L.W. Diggs, whose dedication, perseverance, and energy helped him to shape and further their development. Like those stories, this book is the result of false starts, uneven developments, and unknown trajectories, along with the desire to present Diggs's contribution to medicine as accurately as possible. To this end, I am indebted to many people who helped me in various ways.

The research that yielded this book began as a dissertation in the Department of History at the University of Memphis with the encouragement of my advisor Charles Crawford. His mentorship shaped my work and made the journey of completing this compelling project much easier.

The guidance of several other historians at the University of Memphis also proved invaluable. Aram Goudsouzian enlarged my understanding of twentieth-century America, especially the black experience and the Civil Rights movement, which played such an important role in L.W. Diggs's story and the evolution of the Sickle Cell Center. He saw the value of this project and encouraged me to continue with the research. Through her reading of portions of the book, Jannan Sherman provided many insights into the writing process. Her encouragement helped to sustain my work. Doug Cupples' knowledge of the history of health care in Memphis provided an essential context for the period of Diggs's career in the city.

Two of Diggs's children, Walter and Alice, were most helpful to me by providing interviews that expanded and filled in my understanding of Diggs. Their recollections of their family life were freely given and most illuminating. Walter's generosity began by donating his father's papers to the University of Tennessee's Health Sciences Historical Collections, which provided the foundation for my work and the future work of others.

In addition to the Diggs Collection at the University of Tennessee Health Science Center, a number of archives at various institutions were extremely helpful. The University of Memphis Special Collections Curator Ed Frank gave advice and access to the resources of the Special Collections. The archives at Johns Hopkins University and Randolph Macon College provided valuable documents related to Diggs's student years. Wellesley College's archive released helpful information about Beatrice Mosher's student years.

The Memphis Public Library and Information Center's History Department and its manager Wayne Dowdy contributed background information on many issues concerning relevant people and events in Memphis. Wayne's comments on the manuscript helped to improve the quality of the text and are deeply appreciated.

This work is dedicated to my wife Valeria, whose daily words of encouragement and empathy helped inform this book. Her comments on the manuscript gave it the perspective and understanding of an exceptionally intelligent nonscientist. And to my son Alexander, who often reminded me in his own way of the importance of gaming as a part of the work process. I could not have completed this work without them.

Introduction

> To be a man—clean, strong, happy, honest, truthful, hard working, human—worthy of the respect of other men, and of the love of a real woman—willing to give, restless for growth, and rearing to go.
>
> To become master in Internal Medicine and a teacher willing to work thru lean years for the sake of the cultivation of the art of practice and the advancement of the science of my profession.
>
> To use my time better, allowing space for relaxation, physical exercise, and social enjoyment.
>
> To be *thorough*, systematic, and satisfied c[um] nothing half way done.
>
> —Lemuel W. Diggs, December 1928

The central tenets of Lemuel Whitley Diggs's life were formed as a young man when he began writing down what he considered the most essential attributes of the man he wanted to be. In an early version of his credo written about 1924 and entitled "My Idea of a MAN," his ideal "treats all women with respect and endeavors to protect them from wrong and degredations [*sic*]," respects other people, "loves children and men, horses, dogs, birds, and trees," controls himself, takes care of his body, never quits, and is strong and gentle. In this same entry, he also wrote that a man "is willing to fight for what he loves and is two-fisted." However, in a marginal note dated November 1924, he amends this attribute: "Not so sure, but that a bigger man can accomplish same ends without fighting." By May 1, 1923, while a student at Johns Hopkins University School of Medicine, he called his essential attributes "My Ambitions" and sharpened his focus to include becoming "a great doctor, not a famous one, to know more than any other man about my line in order to give my patients the greatest possibility of recovery" and "to settle in the South and spend my life for the uplift of my country." Here he also inserted an expression of his Virginian and southern upbringing in his desire "to become like [Robert E.] Lee, and like the best of the best men, but not too good to see the best in the worst of men." By December 1928, he had completed a third, and presumably final, version of his ideals just as he was completing his medical training and about to begin his professional career. The only question for the young man would be to determine how his ideals would be translated into his future personal and professional life.[1]

Diggs coveted an academic medical career, one that was idealistic but also grounded in science; he desired to contribute to the progress and growth of the society in which he grew up. His medical career was informed by Jim Crow, the Great Depression, World War II, and the postwar years, and it bears witness to the effects those unstable times had on medicine. This biography is the first narration of the life and career of this physician, researcher, and teacher who accomplished so much and whose influence touched so many.

When Diggs began his career at the University of Tennessee Medical Units in 1929, he was a newly minted academic physician with excellent credentials, eager to launch his career. His medical training took place at Johns Hopkins, which he subsequently capped with a residency at the University of Rochester. He arrived in Memphis as one of the first full-time, paid faculty members at an institution that, like many in the United States at that time, operated almost entirely with volunteers and adjunct faculty from the non-university medical community. Diggs could have chosen private practice for himself with the prospect of building his own practice and earning a substantially better salary, but he preferred the collaborative patient care and research atmosphere of a university setting, the interaction with students and residents, and the opportunity to contribute to the knowledge base of medicine. As an assistant professor, he saw patients at Memphis City Hospital, reviewed their cases, organized the clinical laboratory, and began conducting instructional autopsies for students and residents. Yet, even with the activities of starting a new life and acclimating himself to his new duties, a hint of his future impact on medicine emerged. He immediately recognized that there was an unusually high number of sickle cell patients, a disease that he had been taught was rare. On the speculative assumption that sickle cell anemia might be a metabolic or nutritional disorder, he gave several of the patients whom he saw in the City Hospital a liver extract that he had brought with him from the University of Rochester, which produced no beneficial effect. But this lack of success only deepened the mystery of the disease and initiated his quest to find a cure. He would pursue that goal for the remainder of his life. As Diggs himself explained, "There was always a stimulus to continue the research because the patients had recurring, painful episodes requiring hospitalization and because of the handicapping nature of the hereditary anemia."[2] The young, white physician selected this black disease to be his life's calling for its scientific value, despite the lack of financial or professional encouragement for pursuing research that might lead to a cure.

Diggs's initial thinking was that sickle cell might yield to the concentrated attention of scientific research, but it quickly became clear to him that the illness, with its painless skin ulcers often on the legs, joint pain, the excruciatingly painful episodes known as crises, and its curious sickle-shaped red blood cells, would resist any easy understanding. The symptoms were too varied in his patients to produce an underlying theory of the disease. Over the years, he would discover details about the mechanism of the disease that would hint at ways to ameliorate it, but never that final detail that could yield a remedy. Eventually, sickle cell's resistance to any cure would lead Diggs to expand his thinking beyond the disease in his individual patients to include treating sickle cell as a familial and social concern, rather than simply as an individual one. He was an unusual research-oriented physician who cared about the suffering of his patients as much as he did for the focus of his research.

Upon Diggs's arrival, the University of Tennessee Medical Units was a growing, eighteen-year-old medical school located in the modern southern city of Memphis. Its largely adjunct faculty taught a lively student body of about seven hundred. Graduates of its programs had a reputation as solid clinicians, in part because of their exposure to advanced, and often complex, medical conditions at the Memphis City Hospital. Diggs brought a new way of thinking to an institution that at the time placed little emphasis on research; indeed, research was not considered essential for promotion through the academic ranks. Teaching and clinical service defined the scientific culture in Memphis.

Although he was a faculty member, Diggs worked and saw patients in the Memphis City Hospital, which was a city agency charged with providing healthcare services to the citizens of Memphis; in reality, this meant that it served mainly poor and black people. At any given time, the patient population of the City Hospital was approximately 80 percent black and 20 percent white, and the wards were segregated. This arrangement provided the city an inexpensive and professionally trained medical staff and, in exchange, the university received access to the range of patients and hospital services that were necessary for physician training. The City Hospital was the only hospital in town that would accept black patients, and, in the racial logic of the day, it was perceived by many as a barrier that protected the white community from the diseases that were believed to be propagated in the black community.[3]

Medical racism was an accepted norm in the scientific community of the time. Many physicians, including those in Memphis, saw the black population as a public health menace because of the high incidence of specific diseases such as syphilis, tuberculosis, typhoid fever, malaria, diphtheria, and scarlet fever. Healthcare personnel may have given black patients the same standard of care as whites, but their clinical judgment could be affected, and they could become abusive when black patients failed or refused to comply with instructions for their care. Racism informed all aspects of working life in the Memphis City Hospital, and the John Gaston Hospital that was built after it.[4]

The UT Medical Units and the Memphis City Hospital were also a reflection of the larger community. Jim Crow laws and attitudes were still firmly entrenched in a city in which the machine politics of the mayor, E. H. Crump, ensured that the status quo remained unchallenged. Public institutions such as the schools, the public library, and the zoo were segregated. However, in Memphis, blacks voted in elections in larger numbers than anywhere else in the South. This was part of a quid pro quo between Mayor Crump's political party machine and the black community. As long as blacks voted in elections for Crump's candidates, they would have greater, though not equal, access to public facilities. Crump was famous for his coercive and dictatorial party-boss political style, which landed him on the cover of national magazines. During the period of his influence, Memphis had the feel of a modern city. Free of its past of yellow fever and malaria epidemics, and with magnolias and flowers lining its streets, the city was nonetheless firmly rooted in a racist past and present.[5]

In keeping with his instinct to advance scientific knowledge and to apply scientific advances, Diggs opened a blood bank at the City Hospital in 1938. He felt that the time had come for drawing, preserving, and transfusing blood on demand and exploited the opportunity at the John Gaston Hospital, which replaced the City Hospital in 1936. Despite some initial concerns from the administration and from some colleagues, the blood bank was a personal and medical success that, within a few years, was emulated by other local hospitals. The war in Europe, with its demand for plasma (the liquid part of blood that remains after all cells have been removed) and other blood products, also shaped this success. From the outset, the policy of the bank required blood units to be segregated by race and that blood be transfused by race only. Given the cultural and popular beliefs about blood and race, the City Hospital administration probably created the policy as nothing more than an extension of existing attitudes. Diggs knew that it was medically unnecessary to segregate blood units, because there was no medically discernable difference between black and white blood. Thus, Diggs and the bank's workers formed an unofficial policy of offering blood of the opposite race to patients with their understanding and permission, and the blood bank continued to operate in this way until "the Jim Crow Law in the blood bank was ignored by mutual consent of all intelligent persons."[6] The blood bank was a stunning personal achievement for Diggs.

Diggs was not an altruist seeking to realize an ideal in the world, but more of a public servant using his talents in his profession. He had a strong social conscience that rejected artificial differences in people, whether racial, economic, or otherwise. He wasn't a "joiner," someone who aligned himself with either social or political groups to advance a particular cause. Instead, he had a strong sense of individual responsibility that guided him in his professional and social life. Early in his career he operated as an individual clinical researcher in collaboration with other physicians with similar interests. By the time the Second World War began, he was already thinking about improvements to his university's organization. Realizing perhaps that changing an existing institution was much more difficult than creating a new one, in 1958 he founded the Sickle Cell Center, structured according to his perceptions about how research in this area should be done. His organizational acumen came from his experience at the university, and from what he learned as a participant in the steering committee to form the new St. Jude Children's Research Hospital.

Diggs's rationale for dealing with racial prejudice in the blood bank was typical of the thinking of a political moderate. He recognized, along with many people, that segregation was a serious problem and that black poverty should be eliminated. At the same time, he knew that the problem was complex and could not be resolved easily. When necessary, he found it more appropriate to sidestep the issue until the reason and good sense of others caught up with him, a strategy that would fail him in the turbulent postwar years. Recognizing that no medical evidence supported the policy of segregating blood by race, Diggs and the staff would comply with the Jim Crow policy except in cases where the patient's life was at risk and the necessary black or white blood was unavailable.

Opening the blood bank was a turning point in Diggs's career because it led to his recognition as a local and national expert on blood banking and its uses. Not only for the war effort but for local and regional disasters the need for a blood bank was apparent, but even as this fact was recognized, the lack of funding at the University of Tennessee and the City Hospital made it harder and harder to purchase blood and new equipment as well as to keep up with the growing demand for blood products.

As Diggs's reputation grew, he became frustrated by his slow advancement through the academic ranks, along with the accompanying lag in compensation. At this time promotion was perfunctory, and it is probable that he was promoted to associate professor as a matter of course, but his salary did not increase enough to comfortably support a family with three children. In part, this was due to the effects of the Great Depression, but it also stemmed from the university's shoestring budget, which remained in effect even as the war progressed. Moreover, Diggs began to feel increasingly drawn to the evolving specialty of clinical pathology, an interest his department chair did not share. The war years brought new demands: the university's focus shifted to accommodate demands for educating health-care professionals and for conducting research as dictated by the needs of the armed forces in the European and Pacific theaters. As a result, Diggs conducted research in tropical diseases, including travel to Guatemala and El Salvador, where he had the opportunity to observe the practice of medicine and the social conditions in those cultures.

The war suppressed nearly all activity in sickle cell research. As the war progressed, the total number of papers published nationally on the disease declined annually to one or none. What did appear in print were case reports, offering little that was new. Diggs conducted some research for the U.S. Air Force with regard to black airmen possessing the sickle cell trait and their suitability for flying at high altitudes.

The dearth of new publications and opportunities for research made these years difficult for Diggs. He told colleagues at the University of Tennessee that he wanted more experience with clinical pathology, but his family knew that his decision also had to do with his stagnant salary. He accepted an offer to supervise the clinical laboratory at the Cleveland Clinics in January 1945, where he could do what he enjoyed in a setting that was more in harmony with his professional inclinations. Although the work suited him very well and he thoroughly enjoyed the challenge of working with new people and new methods, the colder northern climate did not agree with his family, which had increased to include a fourth child. At the same time, there was a growing call for him to return to Memphis. His colleagues and patients missed him, and his absence was felt. In 1947, he and the family were able to escape the North for the sunnier climate in Memphis, and he returned with a salary increase and a promotion to full professor.

After World War II, researching and treating sickle cell anemia in the United States grew much more complicated, which challenged the sense of moderation that Diggs relied on for dealing with complex problems. He began to develop an idea of a center that would serve to combine resources and personnel to concentrate on finding a solution to the disease's mystery. Financial help from sources in Memphis to support research became available as early as 1954, many years before funding would become available from the National Institutes of Health. With these limited resources, Diggs created the first sickle cell center in the country in 1958.

The civil rights movement was growing and in unexpected ways made the task of building the new center both easier and harder. Easier federal funding for sickle cell centers around the country did not become available until 1971, which finally allowed Diggs to take advantage of the work already done by him and his staff to expand the personnel and pursue new ideas. As the public perception of medicine became affected by rancorous debate over national health insurance, the rising cost of healthcare, and the ugly revelations of medical scandals—such as the forty-year Tuskegee Syphilis Project, which came to light in 1972—mistrust and suspicion of the federal government loomed over the Sickle Cell Center, which led to questions about what was really taking place there. It was rumored that one of the center's staff members was a spy for a local church organization. These and other related issues contributed a great deal of frustration to Diggs's everyday activities. It was no longer sufficient to wait for cooler heads to prevail, and so Diggs began taking a more active stance on the social issues of the day.

One of the notable successes for Diggs began in 1955, when he was asked to represent the Memphis and Shelby County Medical Society on a steering committee to organize a new pediatric hospital. The idea for this hospital was the brainchild of a Hollywood entertainer, Danny Thomas, who proposed Memphis as the incarnation of his dream. Although the idea for a new children's hospital was initially accepted by city political and medical leaders, it ran into resistance from leaders in the medical community, who questioned the need for an additional facility that would compete with existing pediatric facilities. On Diggs's recommendation, *research* on catastrophic childhood illnesses became the key component of the hospital's support and mission and is reflected in the name, the St. Jude Children's Research Hospital. In effect, St. Jude was the embodiment of one of Diggs's core principles: to have a hospital like no other, where medical research was linked inseparably to patient care, and the operation and cost of the hospital were both supported locally. It was due to Diggs's influence that patients would be accepted into St. Jude programs regardless of race, religion, or financial status.

Blood Picture: L.W. Diggs and Sickle Cell Disease seeks to recall Diggs's life as a physician and an intellectual, as someone who valued personal responsibility and the improvement of medicine and his country. The dramatic progress in twentieth-century American medicine and the turbulent, sometimes clamorous changes in American society were refracted through his life. He pushed the limits of medicine against the existing social state of affairs for patients with sickle cell anemia, sought to implement better healthcare, and spoke out against racist policies in Memphis in public venues. The kind of faith in progress Diggs possessed can be captured in historian Eric Hoffer's comment on progressivism: "Even the sober desire for progress is sustained by faith—faith in the intrinsic goodness of human nature and in the omnipotence of science."[7] Diggs had that kind of faith. With a moderate's sensibility for social justice, Diggs used his professional expertise and authority to navigate the rocky waters of social and medical racism and the civil rights movement of the twentieth century. He transferred the fervor of his Methodist upbringing to leading a moral and meaningful life in pursuit of a cure for sickle cell anemia. Understanding Diggs's life tells us about the consciousness of the South, the power and possibility of American ideals, the ongoing interplay between healthcare and society, and the evolution of the American imagination.

I will be eminent.

—Henry Wadsworth Longfellow, 1824

Chapter 1
A Young Doctor Comes to Memphis

At five feet ten inches tall, Lemuel Whitley Diggs was athletic, self-aware, and confident in his abilities and in the future. He was born in 1900 in Hampton, Virginia, the son of devout Methodist parents, and he arrived in 1929 at the end of a long and demanding road of medical training, ready to begin a new life in Memphis. His father, Chaplin Spencer Diggs, owned a grocery store and grew crops that he sold in the store. As a boy, Diggs worked in the garden, an enjoyment that he would carry with him wherever he lived. The store made a living for the family but was not as profitable as it could have been, in part because his mother, Ruby Diggs, was a strict Methodist who would not allow the sale of alcohol in the store, a decision that was consistent with their Methodist values but limited how much profit the store could make. At family meetings, religious topics, such as the question of the literal translation of the Bible, were discussed seriously and sometimes passionately. Diggs participated in these discussions and was frustrated at how these family discussions could divide people. He didn't think that these discussions solved any issues. As a young man, Diggs also enjoyed playing sports, including baseball, which his family did not allow him to pursue on Sundays. He could not accept the restraints of Methodism, because his temperament led him to seek another calling that would satisfy his desire for a more certain knowledge that might also improve the situation in the South. Thus, it was probably about this time that he developed a skepticism of religion.

Diggs had a lifelong interest in the founding fathers of Virginia, including Washington and Jefferson, but his interest focused on George Mason, who was an opponent of slavery, the principal author of the Virginia Declaration of Rights of 1776 (which was adopted into the Constitution of Virginia and was also a model for Jefferson's draft of the Declaration of Independence), and an ardent proponent of the Bill of Rights of 1789. In particular, it was Mason's distinction between natural and legal individual rights that Diggs found compelling and that would inform his thinking in future debates on healthcare and national health insurance—a subject in which he would maintain a lifelong interest.[1] He would have definite ideas about what government could and could not do regarding personal liberties, and what individuals should expect from their government.

In 1918, Diggs completed his public education at Hampton High School in a class of thirty-seven. His high scholastic achievement was rewarded at graduation with a scholarship to Randolph-Macon College in Ashland, Virginia, where he began his undergraduate education. That same year Diggs was also given a Classification I by his Selective Service Board. As President Woodrow Wilson began to vigorously portray the war in Europe as a struggle between democracy and autocracy and to stress the need for America to join with its democratic allies, American universities and colleges responded by taking up the cause.[2] At Randolph-Macon, students admonished the administration for its lack of preparedness for the coming struggle.[3] Diggs arrived in the fall of 1918 and spent part of his first semester in this atmosphere until the war's end in November of that same year. He spent four months in Student Army Training Corps at Randolph-Macon, where he also blew "assembly." It is not clear from the yearbook whether Diggs gave the signal for the training core to gather, or if this was perhaps a college prank, but the *Yellow Jacket* college yearbook indicated that this activity earned him the nickname of "Twitley." Even though eligible for the army, he was not called up, nor did he enlist. Soon after the war the training corps was disbanded.[4]

If Diggs was dismayed by family disagreements over the meaning of biblical passages, then it is likely that the many extracurricular activities and the college atmosphere at Randolph-Macon further stimulated his dissatisfaction. Randolph-Macon was a Methodist college situated on an idyllic, spacious campus in the Virginia countryside north of Ashland with a network of curving footpaths linking its buildings. It had an all-male student body closely controlled by the Methodist Church, which required that student education be in strict adherence with the principles of its Bible-based theology. At the same time, when Diggs joined the freshman class, the school was caught between the position of a church requiring stricter adherence to Christian principles and the moral and intellectual disruption from American involvement in World War I. In order to keep undesirable influences from taking over and to maintain their high ideals, the church and college administration exerted greater pressure on the faculty and students to observe campus rules.

The result was a ban on drinking alcohol, dancing, and showing movies on campus. Off-campus dancing events remained front-page news in the student newspaper until the college authorities complained about these as well. According to one historian, the most similar historical disruption was caused by the Civil War in the 1860s when the school resisted attempts to turn it into a military academy. The Spanish-American War of 1898 passed almost unnoticed in campus life. Randolph-Macon maintained its decorum, and student life was generally quiet. Radios were not banned on campus but were rare and discouraged in the dormitories. Activities sponsored by the college that took place off-campus—for example, athletic and debating team events—were well attended. Fraternities were also very popular because they functioned as a social nexus on a campus that otherwise provided few venues for social gathering. Fraternities were allowed to have houses, although members were not allowed to sleep in them. Students were forbidden to have automobiles, requiring them to utilize trams and trains to access the forbidden attractions of Richmond some twenty miles away, which Diggs did on occasion with one of his uncles.[5]

It was the family's intent, probably more from his mother, that Diggs become a Methodist minister, and for this purpose Randolph-Macon College was a hopeful choice for the parents. Diggs immersed himself in college life and took advantage of many of the opportunities that he found. He was on the cabinet of the Young Man's Christian Association for four years and president in his last year, and he was a leader in Bible study classes. But Diggs also participated fully in other aspects of campus intellectual life, including work on the weekly newsletter staff as "Humorous Editor" and on the annual staff. He was a member of the Intercollegiate Debate Team, a Little Faculty member in English, read *King Lear* for the Lovers of Shakespeare Club, was treasurer of the junior class and later president of the senior class, and at about 110 pounds he played end on the college football team. College was an opportunity for him to try out new identities and new ideas, and he immersed himself in as many activities as he could.

He joined the Sigma Phi Epsilon fraternity for his social needs as well as a forensic fraternity and a literary fraternity. He continued his passion for sports by playing on the football team while selecting a major in English literature, which must have satisfied his intellectual curiosity. Samuel Taylor Coleridge was one of his favorite poets. Coleridge would have appealed to Diggs for the colorful and elegant use of language and his invention of many words and phrases. He enjoyed participating on the debating team, where he would learn to argue both for and against the issues of the day. This type of mental activity would serve him well throughout his life as a physician when he would need to be able to make his case in a variety of controversial and sometimes contentious circumstances. Once, while representing the opposing side against the resolution "that England should recognize Ireland as an independent republic," Diggs and his partner R. H. Winn won for Randolph-Macon against its rival Richmond College.[6]

By his second college year he determined that he wanted to be a physician. The yearbook noted that, "As a physician, he will render a genuine service to his fellow-man."[7] Diggs began turning away from Methodism and his family's desire that he become a minister. He was attracted to medicine because the profession enjoyed a marked esteem and because of its scientific nature. The rationality of the scientific method appealed to him, and he saw it as more in keeping with his desire for clear and definite knowledge. He very likely had heard about the reputation of nearby Johns Hopkins University's School of Medicine and selected it for that reason. Medicine had the precision of science, which would have appealed to him after the disenchantment stemming from his family's heated discussions on biblical interpretation, and held the promise of being able to perhaps improve the social situation of the South. He completed his bachelor's degree in 1921 but stayed an extra year at the college to finish his master's degree in English in 1922. He also taught as an instructor in that department. In the spring of 1922, he applied to Johns Hopkins, which accepted him in its medical school in June of that year.[8] The cost of medical school was a challenge for Diggs. He had to borrow money from his family, including an uncle, which he was unable to repay until 1938 due to the intervening Great Depression. But he persevered in his quest to join the ranks of students at Hopkins and to graduate from this fine institution.[9]

However Diggs reasoned it, he could hardly have selected a better school for his future career. Located in Baltimore, Johns Hopkins had served as a model for American medical education in many ways since opening its doors in 1893. It was the medical school that Abraham Flexner used in 1910 as the gold standard for all other schools in the United States in the widely influential report now commonly referred to as the Flexner Report.[10] Hopkins was the first school to require an undergraduate degree for admission, to admit women on an equal basis with men, and to create a residency program as an integral part of medical training where students "lived" in the hospital to better care for and learn from their patients. The towering figure of William Osler as physician-in-chief of the Johns Hopkins Hospital and his distinguished successors set the curriculum for the clinical program in which Diggs was trained. From its inception, Hopkins moved almost immediately to the forefront of medical education in the country and consistently attracted the best faculty and student talents to its programs.[11]

After graduating from Randolph-Macon, Diggs lived at home in Hampton. His application to the medical school was brief, only a page of personal information but including a letter from his chemistry professor at Randolph-Macon, Hall Canter, who attested to Diggs's good work at the college. Along with a request for his courses and grades, he was also asked what works he had read in Latin and whether he could read ordinary French and German, to which he replied, "Yes." His application was unproblematic. In a letter dated June 15, 1922, Diggs was informed of his acceptance along with a request for a deposit on his tuition.[12]

From the time he arrived at Hopkins in 1922, he was challenged by the course work as well as clinical duties. The most immediate change was in his social life. At Randolph-Macon he participated in any number of extracurricular activities in addition to the fifteen or so hours of course credit. In medical school there were no extracurricular activities, the number of course hours increased, and the rigor of these courses was extremely demanding. As Kenneth M. Ludmerer observed, "Such an ascetic existence contrasted markedly with the hedonism of many college students during the Jazz Age and reinforced the public's perception of medicine as a calling."[13] It is likely that Diggs was attracted by this sense of calling, and this attraction led him to transfer his family's desire for him to become a Methodist minister to becoming a physician instead. Diggs's courses were very stimulating, in part because there were no formal lectures in anatomy or in other classes, nor did students work for grades. One anatomy professor was memorable because he would not even let students bring their textbooks to class. In Diggs's own words, "He said he wanted us to have the same thrill as there was in the original dissector."[14]

Diggs loved his classes, but the clinical life of a medical student was demanding and at times filled with drudgery. Clinical duties entailed working long hours and performing numerous simple laboratory, therapeutic, and diagnostic functions, also known as "scut work," tasks relatively easy to learn but which had to be performed repetitively over a period of many months. Students could also be called upon to donate blood and participate in other clinical activities beyond the domain of patient care.[15] Diggs struggled with chemistry but was able to pass all of his other subjects easily. Diggs enjoyed it all, including the summer jobs that allowed him to earn extra money for school. His summer work activities included instruction in chemistry in 1923 at Mount Vernon College in Baltimore; in 1924 he participated in the International Health Bureau's Malaria Survey; and in 1925 he was a camp doctor in Cooperstown, New York.

It was at Johns Hopkins that Diggs's interests in hematology and cell morphology were awakened. While a student, he took courses on medical illustration, bacteriology, and other related subjects that emphasized the role of the microscope as a clinical tool. His class was the first requiring that each student purchase and use his own oil-immersion microscope and keep it available at all times, thus reinforcing its importance for the remainder of his career. Indeed, Diggs's career began at about the same time as the use of the microscope became widely accepted as a clinical tool.[16] He also studied sickle cell and other blood diseases under Dr. John Huck, who was working on the clinical features of sickle cell anemia and was the first to argue that it was transmitted according to Mendelian laws.[17]

In the middle of his medical education, Diggs began keeping two notebooks in which he recorded the moral and professional pearls of wisdom that resonated with him about life and medicine. One contained brief, epigrammatic sayings taken from many different sources about the nature of life and manhood. The second contained quotations about the nature and idealism of medical practice and research. The entries were by poets and writers, such as Robert Frost, Henry Wadsworth Longfellow, George Eliot, and Thomas Carlyle; presidents, such as Woodrow Wilson, Teddy Roosevelt, and Franklin Roosevelt; and scientists and doctors, such as William Osler, William W. Keen, and Oliver Wendell Holmes. The notebooks reflect Diggs's desire for crystalized statements of key aspects or principles of life, and his love of language, an abiding interest that he carried with him throughout his career. His fascination with language, in words and their definitions, extended even to the creation of new words as new scientific discoveries were made. He recorded pithy statements in a single location, regardless of the source, as indispensable for his view of the world. Mixed in with the words of others are his personal reflections on what the ideals meant to him, on manhood, individual and professional integrity, family, and country. He began collecting these sayings as a medical student and continued doing so through his internship and residency and into his career at the University of Tennessee.

As a student at Randolph-Macon and Johns Hopkins, Diggs would ride a horse, which was practical for those unable to afford an automobile at this time. One day while he was a medical student, a tree limb knocked him off his horse and he suffered a skull fracture. Dr. Alfred Blalock, then a neurosurgical resident at Johns Hopkins, treated him by using a burr to mill a hole in his skull to relieve the pressure of swelling on his brain, saving his life. Both Diggs and Blalock would remember this event many years afterward.[18] Blalock would later develop the shunt that relieved cyanosis in blue baby syndrome, also known as Tetralogy of Fallot, the result of a defect in the wall separating the two ventricles of the heart that allows deoxygenated blood to mix with the oxygen-rich blood ready to be pumped to the body.

Diggs's first teacher at Hopkins was Florence Rena Sabin, who taught the anatomy class that all incoming students had to take and provided instruction on mounting stained and unstained histology microscope slides. Sabin was his ideal teacher and went on to notable positions at other institutions. Hematology was not a subspecialty in medicine at the time; she and her fellow professors were the first hematologists in the country. The first woman full professor at Hopkins, Sabin maintained interests in, among other areas, the lymphatic system, the supravital staining of living blood cells, and the saturation of erythrocytes.[19] "Some of her enthusiasm for hematology and cell morphology must have rubbed off," Diggs wrote.[20] He also studied for a time under the well-known Hopkins medical illustrator, Max Brödel.[21] Brödel would heighten Diggs's appreciation of "seeing" comprehensively, whether the object was a patient or a slide under a microscope. Diggs would later admonish his students, "If you can't draw it, you haven't seen it."[22] He learned early how the grace and beauty of the visual arts could be employed to clarify scientific ideas. In foregrounding the vitally useful role of art in medical education, Diggs would later employ the talents of a Memphis artist, Dorothy Sturm, to draw the morphology of blood cells from microscopic observation for students. Sabin and Sturm were both women, reflecting Diggs's recognition that women are capable and intelligent. He would use their work as contributors to his education and knowledge, and he would encourage and mentor other women during his career to become healthcare professionals.[23]

Another noted professor at Hopkins was Dr. Stanhope Bayne-Jones, who conducted a memorable course in bacteriology emphasizing the examination of stained and unstained preparations of body fluids. Drs. Paul W. Clough and John G. Huck taught a laboratory course referred to locally as "Clinical Mike" because of the emphasis that was placed on the use of the microscope for patient care. "I remember making drawings of sickled red cells and abnormal cells in other types of anemia," Diggs would recall.[24] Class notes by Diggs from these and other courses contain marginal anatomical drawings in colored pencil to illustrate the points made in class.[25] The notes are clearly written and legible, and his drawings illuminate the point in his notes.

The reputation of Hopkins as a leading, progressive medical school is reflected not only in its faculty members, but also in its reputation and publications, such as the Flexner Report on medical education during the late nineteenth and early twentieth centuries. This character and influence were probably not lost on Diggs, who had a clear idea early in his life that he wanted to be the best at something; he was probably drawn to Hopkins for these reasons. As his preparation for a medical degree neared an end, he could not have missed noticing the news of a new school of medicine and dentistry being formed at a university in the state of New York. A new school at this time was remarkable news if only because the

Rochester school was being built at a time when the overall number of medical schools in the nation was declining significantly. So many Hopkins faculty members were moving to the new program at Rochester that it was probably on the advice and by the example of his professors that he chose to do an internship and residency at the newly built Strong Memorial Hospital that was part of the University of Rochester. He could have gone into practice with just his medical degree, but he understood that specializing with an internship and residency in pathology and hematology would enhance his future prospects considerably. In addition, two of his professors at Strong Memorial, George Whipple and William McCann, would have appealed to his moderate political sensibilities. Whipple was the revered dean of the medical school at the University of Rochester. He was a respected researcher, but he felt, as did his students, that his highest accomplishment was as a teacher. McCann was the first chair of the Department of Medicine and established the Hematology-Oncology Unit at the University of Rochester.[26]

At the completion of his medical degree in 1926, Diggs did indeed go on to specialized training in pathology at Rochester, which had started its new medical school and opened a new hospital. He was in the first group of about twenty-four young physicians, interns, and residents; in 1928 he became Rochester's first hematologist.[27] He interned for two of his three years under William McCann, who was chair of the Department of Medicine. Here he learned, in his words, "to participate in developing laboratory procedures, stocking clinical laboratories, starting a syphilis clinic and teaching." There were opportunities for him as part of this first group of interns at a new hospital and university, and Diggs seized the chance to learn everything he could. At this time there were no laboratory technicians or medical students to perform basic laboratory tests, so the interns were required to perform all routine tests, including basal metabolism and electrocardiograph tests. In addition, emergency chemical tests had to be done at night and on holidays. Despite the drudgery and monotony, Diggs's decision to specialize in clinical pathology and hematology was reinforced: "Instead of being bored with and resentful of laboratory assignments I became interested in Clinical Pathology and Hematology." After his year as a new intern, he was assigned to the infectious disease unit and the bacteriology and transfusion laboratory. In his third year, a formal Department of Hematology was formed and Dr. McCann assigned him the task of teaching the first course in clinical pathology and hematology to medical students, as well as giving lectures to nurses.[28]

In keeping with his fondness for the linguistic turn, Diggs later recalled the story of George Whipple and William Leslie Bradford from the Department of Pediatrics, who coined the term "thalassemia" (a hereditary form of anemia found chiefly in people of Mediterranean origin) to replace other names by which the disease was known, such as "Mediterranean" or "Cooley's" anemia. Diggs good-naturedly blamed Bradford for "suggesting a seemingly erudite, but less meaningful and less understood Greek word." Bradford and Diggs both played on the Strong Memorial baseball team in Rochester. When asked why he had changed the name of the disease to "thalassemia," Bradford replied, "A good baseball player does not argue with the umpire."[29] Diggs's love of language was essential to his character throughout his life and would sustain him in other debates as new medical knowledge emerged.

It was also while at the University of Rochester that Diggs met Beatrice Moshier, a young woman working in the laboratory who helped feed the dogs beef, liver, skeletal and muscle extracts, and other substances as part of Whipple's ongoing nutritional experiment. She graduated from Wellesley College in 1926, the same year as Diggs from Randolph-Macon College, and returned home to take additional classes at the University of Rochester.[30] A native of Rochester, Beatrice was also employed at the university in Dr. Whipple's "Animal House," where he maintained a colony of dogs that he used in his nutritional studies. It was in this environment that she and Diggs became friends and fell in love; after a courtship, they became engaged to be married. Over the years, they would often repeat the story to friends that, while she was feeding extracts to the dogs, he was feeding extracts to the patients. She was a contrast to Diggs. Her family upbringing and college training made her more liberal and freethinking in her outlook. Her family belonged to the Unitarian Church of Rochester, which captured Diggs's interest, probably due to her influence.[31]

Whipple's nutritional research began around 1918 as an investigation into the difference that specific foods could make in the improvement of anemia. Together with his assistant, Frieda Robscheit-Robbins, Whipple maintained the dog colony as the basis for his research into the role of nutrition in anemia. After Whipple arrived at Rochester in 1921, the first building constructed was the one that came to be known as the "Animal

House." Staff offices were also located there. The dogs would be bled to maintain a known level of red blood cells and would then be fed various foods to see which dogs would replace the lost cells most quickly with which foods. The result was a clear indication that some anemias required nothing more than a nutritional adjustment to bring about an improvement. This turned out to be especially true in the case of the uniformly fatal disease known as "pernicious anemia." In 1934 Whipple received the Nobel Prize in Physiology or Medicine, along with George Richard Minot and William Parry Murphy, for this research. In Diggs's mind, this example of the certain and progressive knowledge that scientific research could produce must have represented a more satisfying world than that of his family's discussions about the interpretation of biblical passages.

Diggs's stimulating experience at the University of Rochester no doubt gave him the additional experience and the training that he wanted. The intellectual atmosphere that Whipple expected of all faculty and staff, involving interactions without regard to rank, together with the encouragement of a high level of intellectual achievement, contributed to Diggs's sense of satisfaction. Diggs observed firsthand Whipple's evenhandedness in his administration of the faculty and students in the wards, during lectures, and in the midst of the inevitable clashes of egos. On one occasion, Diggs's clinical notes on a pending case of erysipelas (an acute streptococcal infection) were criticized: "As a Resident in Medicine assigned to the Infectious Disease Unit, my observations relating to patients receiving the serum were recorded. Serious objection was expressed regarding my clinical notes and my statement that the serum sickness that often developed was worse than the disease. Whipple calmed the troubled waters by stating that 'honest differences of opinion are what make horse races.'"[32] Diggs was very pleased with his three-year experience of as a member of this select group. His satisfaction with the institution and his colleagues is recorded on the back of a group photograph of his Rochester class that was taken in 1927. In the picture he is dressed in a suit and bow tie and wearing round, dark-rimmed glasses. He wrote on the back: "A peach of a crew to work with. Not a loafer or a crab in the outfit."[33]

Diggs recalled that the pinnacle of his training at the University of Rochester came while he participated in a nutritional trial under Dr. George Whipple's supervision to find a cure for pernicious anemia. The onset of this fatal disease was so gradual that patients usually could not remember when they first noticed the symptoms. The characteristic manifestations included the triad of a sore mouth or glassy-appearing tongue, a slight jaundice of the eyes and skin, and numbness or tingling of the fingers or toes. The disease could also lead to a demyelinating lesion of the spinal cord, leading to personality and memory changes that could only be visualized in an autopsy. At the heart of the disease was a mysteriously declining red cell count. Whipple's experimentation on dogs gave the first indication that liver extract could reverse the decline in red blood cells and resolve the disease's symptoms. This research into the correlation between foods and anemia started in the animal house and progressed from there to humans. The clinical use of humans investigated the response in patients to different extracts of liver, kidney, spleen, and bone marrow. A range of dietary supplements had been tried at other institutions, with mixed results, and it was clear that only some supplements showed promise. Whipple had already established that liver extract seemed to hold the key. Diggs would later observe that Whipple's work had "proved that 'Popeye' was wrong about the virtues of spinach," and that "the Dairy Council had overstated the value of milk as a complete food."[34] For him it was an example of the power of science to improve health and well being.

Diggs had been assigned to grind liver extract for his patients, one of whom refused to take the extract due to her mental deterioration. The decision was made to force-feed her by inserting a gastric tube instead of giving her a transfusion. Over a period of days Diggs monitored her blood count, hemoglobin, and reticulocyte (immature red cell) counts, and the response could not have been more dramatic. As Diggs recalled, "The transformation of this terminally sick and maniacal patient in a few days' time with the megaloblastic [abnormally large, immature, and dysfunctional red blood cell] cells disappearing from her blood smears and the erythrocyte values steadily increasing was probably the high light [*sic*] of my medical experience. It proved to me the value of basic and applied research."[35] More than just the personal satisfaction that he felt at helping a patient recover from what otherwise would have been a fatal outcome, Diggs believed that this experience memorably characterized the rationalism and methodology of science as the key to producing more such therapies for intractable illnesses.

Despite this clinical success and the breakthrough it seemed to represent, a complete conquest of pernicious anemia would continue to remain elusive. Some patients with a clear diagnosis of the disease still failed to respond to the liver extract, and a remission in the disease was almost certainly followed by one or more relapses. Once the liver extract had been identified as a cure for the disease, Eli Lily & Co. began producing its Liver Extract 343. Scientific medicine and the drug companies were positioning themselves to bring even greater benefits. Nevertheless, the cure reversed the perception of the disease as uniformly fatal, which gave the appearance of conquering the disease.[36]

With his training at an end, it was time for Diggs to find a medical center where he could begin his career, and a community he could settle in to begin a new life with his fiancée. He had the sensibilities of a researcher and a clinician, and he undoubtedly wanted an institution that would allow him to continue his work. He also had a strong desire to return to the South. A medical center associated with a university would suit him best. In the spring of 1929, Diggs visited the chair of the Pathology Department, also a Hopkins graduate, on the campus of the University of Tennessee Medical Units in Memphis. Since he had this opportunity, he decided to plan his visit to include the Kentucky Derby in early May, where Clyde van Dusen won easily that year. He could stop and enjoy the race on his way home. According to Alfred Paul Kraus, "Diggs had always wanted to see the Kentucky Derby. . . . He recalls that it was fortunate that he had his return ticket from Louisville to Rochester since he 'was way ahead until the last race.'"[37] Since they were engaged, Beatrice did not accompany him on this trip. She had stayed behind in Rochester while he went ahead to work and to make preliminary arrangements for their home.

The interview trip to Memphis must have impressed Diggs both in light of the professional prospects for himself and of the location for a home with his fiancée. Harry C. Schmeisser was the chair of the Department of Pathology and Bacteriology at this time. He came from Emory University after a seven-year period as a student and instructor at Hopkins. The administrative officer of the medical units, O. W. Hyman, recalled that Schmeisser "brought to Memphis a clear conception of what should be done to develop a first-class Department of Pathology and Bacteriology, and during the next several years was able to supplement the staff and rearrange the work so that by the time he had been in Memphis five years, the University had a good Department of Pathology."[38] Schmeisser came to Memphis in 1921 and in the intervening years helped to develop a strong

Department of Pathology, which no doubt influenced Diggs's decision to join the department. Schmeisser had a reputation of being a good teacher on the wards to the residents, but he was terrible in the classroom, where he often preferred to just read from textbooks to the students rather than delivering prepared lectures.[39]

For medical schools in general, pathology as a specialty grew slowly in the first half of the twentieth century. It was one of the basic scientific departments that performed autopsies for educational, medical, and research purposes and which came to include bacteriological and histopathological studies, especially cancer. Autopsies were often the only way that diseases could be confirmed or definitively diagnosed. They were also often the first step in finding an underlying cause for a new or mysterious disease. The clinical-pathological conference (CPC), with its regularly scheduled autopsies, was a familiar feature in medical schools and an important teaching forum. During these conferences, autopsies would be performed with students, interns, and residents observing the procedure, with the expectation that observers would visualize the lesions and then think about them in terms of the pathological anatomy at the patient's bedside. In 1926, the American College of Surgeons required accredited hospitals to hire qualified pathologists and perform diagnostic tests and autopsies. This new requirement probably played a role in Schmeisser's need for a full-time pathologist to be placed in the university's main teaching hospital, the Memphis City Hospital.[40]

In May, Diggs had received a letter from Dr. Schmeisser offering him a position as assistant professor of pathology: this was the university's first full-time faculty position in the Department of Medicine. Diggs sent his acceptance of the position, and just three days later Dr. Schmeisser drafted a short, enthusiastic letter of acknowledgment: "Your letter of May 20th accepting appointment of Assistant Professor of Pathology was received with genuine pleasure by us all."[41] On the same day, Schmeisser also sent a more formal letter to the dean of the College of Medicine, Thomas Palmer Nash, requesting Diggs's appointment at an annual salary of $4,000. This was a median-range, entry-level salary at a time when salaries for an assistant professor ranged from $1,050 to $8,000.[42] At one of the leading medical schools, a researcher's salary might be worth as much as $15,000. This letter was pro forma, but it listed the details of Diggs's training and his duties teaching the clinical microscopy course, as well as supervising the clinical laboratories. Graduating from Hopkins and studying under Drs. Whipple and McCann made Diggs a valuable addition to the University of Tennessee Medical Units. It probably made the decision easier for Schmeisser to select Diggs, because he had also graduated from Hopkins seventeen years earlier and knew what this prestigious school would bring to his program. Equally important, the letter touted Diggs's postgraduate training under two internationally respected physicians, William S. McCann and George H. Whipple, at the University of Rochester.

Our main business is not to see what lies dimly
at a distance, but to do what lies clearly at hand.
—Thomas Carlyle

Chapter 2

Memphis

From its inception in 1911, the University of Tennessee Medical Units operated on a shoestring budget from the Tennessee State Assembly that included a small compensation component for
faculty, with the result that its administration relied almost exclusively on
volunteer and part-time faculty. Financial support for the campus stemmed
primarily from state allocations, clinical fees, and student tuition. Although
local physicians could earn far more in private practice, many were willing
to forgo some of the financial compensation of private practice in favor
of the prestige associated with a university appointment. Practicing physicians were attractive to universities because of the accepted idea that they,
not the full-time faculty members, possessed the appropriate kind of clinical experience and knowledge for training and educating students. This
made it possible for the medical school to have skilled, inexpensive adjunct
practitioners on its faculty. In contrast, full-time faculty, it was felt, might
get lost in the ivory tower where their clinical skills would dull, and this,
in turn, make them poor teachers. Academic physicians usually spent part
of their time in clinics and in patient care, but only those fully engaged
in the practice of medicine were considered suitable instructors. Despite

this controversy, pressure increased for medical schools nationwide to begin maintaining a full-time faculty dedicated to staying current with the growth of medical knowledge and innovation. Diggs's appointment grew out of this trend for the Medical Units by virtue of being one of the few full-time faculty appointments on the campus, and the first in the Department of Medicine.

The University of Tennessee Medical Units opened in July of 1911. The State of Tennessee provided minimal funding to create the campus in Memphis. At the same time, the University of Tennessee was keen on having a medical school affiliated with it. The roots of the Memphis campus extend back as far as 1876, when the University of Tennessee in Knoxville established a loose affiliation with the University of Nashville Medical College. The UNMC, a proprietary school, gained the right to display the University of Tennessee name on its diplomas while, at the same time, the University of Tennessee could add a medical school to its programs. UNMC kept the fees it collected for both cost and profit, and UT provided no resources or faculty to the medical school's operation. When the school was transferred to Memphis in 1911 and operating costs were assumed by the Knoxville campus, it is unlikely that either the University of Tennessee nor the Tennessee State Assembly understood how much it would cost to start and maintain a medical school, including the number of faculty needed or the amount and cost of scientific equipment required for training physician-scientists. According to James Hamner, "The unvisionary Tennessee State Legislature would only appropriate paltry funds for the University, making even minimal improvements in the facilities, library, teaching aids, and faculty salaries difficult. Therefore, the University depended in no small measure mostly on either voluntary or part-time faculty."[1] Medical training was, and still is, a more labor-intensive activity than other forms of higher education. The ratio of faculty to students is lower, and the need for equipment and appliances for laboratories and hospitals is higher. It is possible that the state's lack of understanding of these issues was built into the genes of the campus as a continuing, perennial problem.[2]

Diggs's grew up in the pre–World War I era, characterized by Teddy Roosevelt and the dynamism of an emerging national pride in a country that saw itself as a beacon to the world and a democratic model to emulate and expand across the globe. In that spirit, Diggs's goal was to be the best that he could be as a man and a physician, and not to waste a single moment in the achievement of both. He was practical and frugal in the way in which he conducted his life and his professional activities—a characteristic that was probably learned at home, but which was emphasized while he was under the influence of George Whipple at the University of Rochester.[3] His medical education took place at a time when patient care and research were at the center of medical education; culturally, doctors were considered heroes and part of a fraternity dedicated to helping the sick through the application of science. By the time Diggs entered medical school, the three principles of patient care, research, and education were firmly established in the leading medical schools as essential to the practice of modern medicine and would continue as canonical throughout the twentieth century.

Diggs came of age at a time when Jim Crow was the established social norm, and in an age that advocated Social Darwinism. It is noteworthy that this was a time before the civil rights movement, feminism, and a healthy skepticism of corporations' involvement in healthcare. Diggs's arrival in Memphis took place only a few months before the Stock Market Crash of 1929, which would signal an economic tsunami making its slow and threatening way to Memphis.

He was looking for a job and found one in Memphis. His ambition to achieve something in his life allowed him to consider the city as his new home at a time when few Virginians chose to move there.[4] Along with his new appointment, he was scouting for a house to rent, where he and his fiancée Beatrice could live. They were planning their wedding at the same time that they were contemplating their move. One phase of Diggs's life was now completed, and he was eagerly looking forward to the next one.

As a medical center and a modern city with a reputation for being clean and progressive, Memphis was a good choice for Diggs. But that reputation grew out of a darker period in the city's history. In the early years of the nineteenth century, the swampy territory on the banks of the Mississippi provided an excellent location for the riverfront settlement that later came to be know as Memphis. But the very landscape that gave Memphis its ideal commercial location would also be the source of a public-health nightmare. The warm, humid summers known as the "sickly season" provided a rich environment for epidemics and other health problems, including dengue, smallpox, and cholera. As the city grew into a transportation hub, diseases from riverboats traveling up and down the Mississippi River brought illnesses from other parts of the country. People remembered the muddy streets and the accumulation of human excrement due to the lack of any public sanitation. The city managed well during the Civil War. It was a major hub for Union activities, including an unprecedented growth in the number of hospitals and medical teams for soldiers in the thousands of military confrontations that took place in Tennessee and Mississippi. At the same time, many Memphians fled to escape the Union occupation and non-Memphians streamed to the city in search in search of safety from the raging war.[5] After the war, the number of doctors and pharmacists grew in proportion to the population growth, and so did medical societies and schools.

The city suffered major health problems during the course of the century, but nothing affected or defined Memphis more than the yellow fever epidemics of the 1870s. "Yellowjack," as it was also known, struck the city throughout the nineteenth century and, before 1870, it took the lives of a few hundred people each time. Before the 1870s, it was even said that the epidemics that struck Memphis were relatively light compared to other locations—that is, until the epidemics of 1873 and 1878, when the disease struck the town with a fury that devastated its population and reputation, and altered its political future. In 1873, over 2,000 people died, and in 1878 a total of 5,150 people succumbed. In January of 1879 the city lost its charter, and the Board of Health was formed with almost dictatorial powers to deal with the health problems of the city.[6]

If there was a silver lining for Memphis, it was that sanitation became an issue of paramount importance. The fear that grew from the yellow fever attacks of the 1870s focused attention on preventing any recurrence by cleaning up the city and installing a sanitation system. According to Memphis historican Patricia LaPointe McFarland, "The city, which had been humiliated by the calamity of the yellow fever epidemics and made the object of national concern was extremely anxious to remedy its unhappy reputation as one of the most unsanitary cities in the country."[7] In 1880, construction began on a new sewer system that took seven years to install. Although yellow fever would continue to be diagnosed in the city for decades, the number of cases was small enough to help the city maintain its focus on sanitation and cleanliness. Together with water-closet construction and street cleaning, the change to Memphis counted as a transformational accomplishment that did much to create its new image as a modern city in the twentieth century.[8]

* * *

Lemuel Whitley Diggs arrived in Memphis during the first days of September 1929, a period of hot, humid, and partly cloudy weather. He had come to begin the duties of his first professional appointment as an assistant professor of pathology. His arrival marked not only the advent of his professional career; he had become engaged to Beatrice Mosher and was ready to begin his new life with her. Memphis represented a promising setting for Diggs to begin his career. According to the 1930 U.S. census, the growing city had a population of approximately 253,140, an increase of 56 percent over the previous census. Of this number, 61.8 percent were white and 38.1 percent black.[9] In 1929 Memphis, as the largest city in Tennessee, had expanded to include 20.3 square miles of suburban land. Its population had become relatively homogeneous as a result of the yellow fever epidemics of the 1870s, and this trend continued into the twentieth century. Moreover, the city's population swelled as part of the national migration from the countryside to the city at the turn of the century; the city was also a stopping point for many migrants from the South to the North in the years after World War I. Memphis had problems with crime and segregation, but it also had a reputation as a progressive southern city, due in large measure to the city's notorious party organizer and boss Edward Hull Crump.[10] E. H. Crump was not mayor when Diggs arrived in Memphis, nor did he hold any elective office. He was the head of a political organization that had dominated city politics for decades. Those in office at this time, including the current mayor, Watkins Overton, were there because of Crump's backing.

Although Crump generally took little interest in the administration of the Memphis City Hospital, he nevertheless had an interest in addressing public-health issues. In his first term as mayor, Crump appointed a well-known local physician, Max Goltman, as superintendent of the Memphis Health Department, who served from 1910 to 1914. During this time, the Health Department began the regulation of the milk industry, which required dairies to be clean and their cows to be free of infection with bovine tuberculosis. The Board of Health authorized school teachers to inspect children for symptoms of contagious diseases, and they could be fined if they allowed a child to return to school without a doctor's certificate. Midwives were required to take an examination to receive a license to practice.

As a Tennessee congressman in the U.S. House of Representatives, Crump introduced a bill to increase funds to public health agencies combatting malaria in the Mississippi Valley. According to G. Wayne Dowdy, "City agencies became adjuncts to Crump's congressional office; the health department, for example, sent a weekly list of all newborn babies to the congressman's office, which then mailed a government publication on child care to their parents."[11] As a Progressive Era politician, Crump could see the value of public health to his career and to his party machine.

Memphis was a southern city in the sense that nearly all of its citizens were either born in Memphis or in other southern states.[12] In the words of one historian, "These recent arrivals from the country-side who were responsible for giving the city a decidedly provincial air included in their cultural baggage such items as a nostalgic devotion to the southern Lost Cause, a propensity for violence, and belief in stringent codes of honor, fundamentalist religion, and white supremacy."[13] Memphis was the nation's largest inland cotton market, and it remained a one-crop town with a very small textile industry. The city also included the University of Tennessee Medical Units and a mix of private hospitals, with the Memphis City Hospital serving as the only public hospital that predominantly served the poor and African American patients.

One of the early questions that Lemuel Diggs and his wife, Beatrice, were often asked after arriving in Memphis was, "Which church will you attend?" Memphis had Methodist, Presbyterian, and Episcopal churches throughout the nineteenth century, but by the turn of the twentieth century it could be said that the city generally adhered to Protestant fundamentalism.[14] As one historian put it, "If cotton dominated the economic life of Memphis and the Delta, religion dominated its social life."[15] Beatrice was a Unitarian Universalist, and Diggs had been raised in a strict Methodist family. If Diggs was something of an outsider by virtue of his education, then his religion further enhanced that perception. The Unitarian Church in Memphis at this time was one of the smallest in the city. The seed of change for Diggs was probably planted at home in Hampton with the family's sometimes contentious discussions, but the transformation for him began while he was a medical student, and accelerated when he met Beatrice at the University of Rochester. He still referred to himself as Methodist, something his chair believed, probably as way of protecting his privacy, but Diggs chose Unitarian Universalism as more compatible with his own thinking personally and scientifically. The couple decided to join the congregation of the First Unitarian Church in Memphis, stewarded by Reverend John Petrie, who maintained the practice of an open pulpit where anyone could speak. Diggs was dissatisfied with the religious discussions he remembered from his family reunions and was no doubt partially influenced by the deism that was popular among colonial leaders. Thus, while still a student at Randolph Macon and later at Johns Hopkins, he gradually moved away from his family's Methodist roots to embrace a faith tradition that would be more open and compatible with his own views.

Beatrice's came from an East Coast liberal family that was part of the Unitarian tradition for several generations. Her mother attended a Unitarian church in Rochester, New York, where Susan B. Anthony taught Sunday school, and she was related to Anthony by marriage. Her mother set high standards for etiquette and honesty.

As a child, Beatrice overcame polio, but she also "attended a pioneering woman's canoeing camp in Canada where there was and is no hot water,"[16] which she loved. She later graduated from Wellesley College. An uncle discovered a modern process for making vinegar from apples, and the financial success of this discovery allowed her to afford a very good liberal arts education. She would later be described as an old guard Rockefeller Republican, but frugal and even businesslike in her family life, and not a materialist. She enjoyed farming as much as Diggs did, and was able to wring a chicken's neck. For years the family kept a cow, which she and her second son milked, and she boiled the milk. Her religious convictions probably influenced her husband to become Unitarian. Both Diggs and his wife would have felt uncomfortable in some of the stricter and more fundamentalist churches in Memphis. The Unitarian Universalist Church's theology contained, in addition to an openness of faith, an intellectual component that appealed to Diggs, especially the reliance on one's own ability to reason. All of these considerations played a role in the young couple's decision to join the Unitarian Church in 1930.[17]

During his first years in Memphis, Diggs acclimated himself to his new setting as an academic physician. He wanted to develop an understanding of the patients he would see, as well as become acquainted with his new colleagues. Only one important order of business remained, and that was his wedding to Beatrice Moshier. On October 18, 1930, they exchanged vows in Rochester, where her family was. The chair of the Department of Pathology, Harry Schmeisser, loaned the newlyweds his vacation house, called Chestnut Lodge, in Blowing Rock, North Carolina, an idyllic, wooded area where the couple could spend a secluded honeymoon. By this time Diggs had rented a home for the couple in Hawthorn Street, about two miles from the Memphis City Hospital.[18] As rents rose, they also lived on Evergreen and Washington streets until 1938 when Diggs completed re-paying his student loan. They saved their money and were able to build a single-family house on five acres of land that they purchased on Farrow Road in White Haven. The house was located in what was then a semirural area about ten miles from the university. By the time it was built, there were three children: Walter, born in 1932, Alice in 1934, and John in 1936. The land also provided room to grow a good-sized garden. Once a year they would hire a local African American to plow the garden. They would raise corn, tomatoes, butter beans, string beans, and other vegetables. Diggs would do the planting, and Beatrice would do the picking. The garden was not unlike the one he worked in to provide vegetables for his family's store. He did not accept memberships to men's organizations; instead he called the garden his country club. The extra room on their property also provided space to have cookouts and for the children to play.[19]

Diggs's move to Memphis, followed by his marriage the next year, represented a happy period of his life. Like other white citizens of Memphis, he remained relatively untouched for months by the economic troubles slowly making their way across the country. He was earning a reasonably good salary, and he had the chance to establish himself and his career as a doctor and member of a university faculty. There was some question about just how important all of the noise emanating from the eastern financial centers could possibly be. It is customary to mark the beginning of the Great Depression with the Stock Market Crash in 1929, but it took about a year for the economic effects to reach the Bluff City because of the distribution and service character of its economy. Indeed, in October of 1929, the gloomy financial news affected only a few downtown speculators. The two daily newspapers carried no headlines of financial disaster or suicide. The *Memphis Commercial Appeal* reported on rumors of a major national disaster as "unbelievably silly" and generously quoted President Hoover on the nation's good health."[20] Despite the local confidence, however, by the time of the Diggs's marriage in 1930 the optimistic mood in Memphis had changed.

As industry began to slow, cotton prices dropped and traffic on the Mississippi River slowed to a trickle. Unemployment rose dramatically, overwhelming the city's public relief services.[21] In 1931 the Tennessee state legislature reduced employee salaries in the Medical Units by 10 percent in January and then again by 9 percent in July. Diggs's promised salary dropped from $4,000 to $3,240, but he was lucky to have continuing employment.[22] The advice offered by the Hoover administration declared that the country was on sound economic footing. In time, Hoover believed, market forces would identify the source of economic instability, which he believed lay outside the United States and, once identified, the market would correct itself. As one historian noted concerning the scene in Memphis, "The increasing frequency of suicides served as a grim barometer of the worsening situation. Suddenly so many people were jumping off Harahan Bridge into the Mississippi that the newspapers printed the names and telephone numbers of clergymen and urged the dispirited to seek counseling. 'Soon a Memphis preacher jumped off.'"[23] Although perhaps apocryphal, the image of people jumping off a bridge illustrated the sense of desperation felt by thousands of unsuccessful job seekers in the region. By early 1932 the economic situation in the country was perceived as dire. Nevertheless, the delay in Memphis's economic decline in 1930 allowed the Diggs family to settle into their new situation and begin to plan for their future.

There were changes slowly taking place in Memphis medicine as a more scientific culture formed. Diggs had been trained in the new model of the physician-scientist, one who was comfortable in the clinic caring for patients and in the laboratory performing tests and carrying out research based on this connection. For him, these activities represented two sides of the same coin: his patients and their illnesses were his laboratory, while the laboratory was where he learned about his patients and their diseases.[24] Scientific knowledge and his own research were mediated by his clinical judgment to help his individual patients. His clinical research would focus on finding ways to improve treatments for various diseases, and would likewise be informed by what he learned from his patients. Diggs's heroes were the medical faculty at Johns Hopkins University, who taught and practiced in the tradition of William Osler. It was there that he began to appreciate pathology and the growing field of hematology. At the University of Rochester and the Strong Memorial Hospital, his heroes were the school's dean, George Whipple; its first chief of medicine, William McCann; and the second chief of pediatrics, William Bradford. Under McCann, Diggs taught the university's first course in hematology. He brought the training he had received and the ideals instilled in him to his new career in Memphis.[25]

William Osler established the training of all medical students coming through Hopkins. Before he left, Osler hand-picked his successor to ensure that the traditions he established would be faithfully maintained. All students, he believed, should receive their clinical instruction beginning with the patient, and their training should likewise end with the patient. His approach to the laboratory was much the same: all research began with the medical literature and ended by contributing to it. The literature, consisting of books and journals, was the bedrock of medical research and understanding; the high-quality training Diggs received as a result of both a patient orientation and reading voraciously in the medical literature contributed to his success.[26] He was also well read outside of medicine, with his degree in English literature from Randolph Macon College.[27]

Diggs drew inspiration from his patients, as his experience with pernicious anemia demonstrated. The potential power of science to alter the course of a life-threatening disease was evident to him. His belief in the laboratory orientation and reliance on the microscope in particular drew him to a blood picture of sickle cell anemia that looked starkly like one he had seen as a student.[28] He knew that the human eye could be very useful in ordinary circumstances, but the microscope was better suited for close observation. He had studied sickle cell anemia while in John G. Huck's clinical microscopy class at Hopkins. He had spent even more time on a similar disease, thalassemia (another hemolytic anemia caused by an inability to synthesize hemoglobin), that was known to be endemic to people in the Mediterranean region. When he saw the elliptical, sickle-shaped cells characteristic of sickle cell anemia, his medical curiosity was piqued.

He knew that little was known about the disease, and as a consequence decided to perform his first, informal laboratory test on it by using the liver extract given to him by Whipple that had been so successful in treating patients with pernicious anemia: "Dr. Whipple gave me some samples of liver extract to test out on people with iron deficiency anemia and pellagra which was then present. But, when I came to Memphis, I came across cases of sickle cell anemia at the old Memphis City Hospital. And, I became so interested in sickle cell anemia." He knew that "nothing was known about the disease hardly at that time."[29] But the liver extract produced no results, and it must have become apparent to him fairly quickly that sickle cell anemia would not yield to a nutritional therapy. He examined his patients in all stages of life, including the "patients at the old folks' home who were over fifty years of age and who remembered slave days and the Civil War."[30] As he pursued sickle cell, the puzzle grew and only deepened his conviction to find a solution. He retained the sense of religious zeal that he had learned at home, and he transferred this sense of dedication to medicine, in particular to solving the mystery of sickle cell anemia.

The microscope was his preferred clinical investigative tool. Its importance was established at Hopkins, where the students in Diggs's class were required to own an oil-immersion microscope. A microscopic view allowed students to see normal cells, but also those that were abnormal and, thus, to see and define the characteristics of individual pathologies. One of Diggs's new duties included teaching microscopy in a course that he dubbed "Clinical Mike." The microscope was no less powerful as a research tool, where the purpose of the endeavor was not so much to benefit an individual patient as to aid in generalizing about the material being enlarged and potentially expanding the scientific knowledge base on sickle cell or other diseases. The microscope, like other technologies, could help to conceptualize the world as mediated by the microscopic image by presenting a world too small to see with the eye alone. By visualizing the microscopic landscape in this way, a level of physical features and objectivity could be achieved that made the production of new knowledge possible[31] Diggs as a clinician and a researcher was the arbiter of what he saw clinically and microscopically, which meant that he could give the subject the clarity and definition that he sought both for himself and for the scientific eye represented by the community of researchers.

His appointment was with the university, but his work would be in the city's public hospital. It was only a few years before, in 1924, that Memphis and the UT Medical Units had entered into an agreement by which the city would supply the nurses, facilities, and patients, while the Medical Units would supply the doctors and medical supplies. The Medical Units did not own a hospital, so this collaboration offered many advantages. In effect, it would give the university an "almost limitless wealth of clinical material afforded by the General Hospital," which would cost nothing to the university and would give it a more-or-less equal status with other medical schools with better endowments.[32] The hospital itself was old by the time Diggs had arrived, but it was a recognized city landmark.

Diggs found himself in this largely favorable administrative arrangement. His office, the laboratory he would use, and the patients he would see were all in close proximity. Diggs's office was located next to the Memphis City Hospital, a sixty-three-year-old building that was the city's only public hospital. He taught classes in the Institute for Clinical Investigation in the warm, humid, and sometimes stifling Memphis climate, which often required keeping the classroom windows open. Some of those windows overlooked Russwood Park, a baseball stadium that was home to the city's minor-league team, the Memphis Chicks, which meant that noise from a game often interfered with classroom instruction. Diggs remembered that one of his toughest assignments was holding the attention of medical students when "the Chicks were in town and the score was tied with a man on third base."[33] It was not an ideal environment and probably the kind of situation that new faculty sometimes have to work through at the beginning of their careers. A colleague also remembered the institute's challenges: "The fact that the other windows faced the nurse's home didn't help any, either."[34]

Diggs represented the cutting edge of medicine for his day. His laboratory-based, research-oriented way of helping patients was a reflection of his training, but it also stood in contrast to the situation he encountered in Memphis. He was out of step with many of the physicians in Memphis, many of whom were home-grown and for whom research was a part of faculty responsibilities, but not encouraged. Diggs recalled: "Patients and physicians, alike, did not support research efforts." But here, at the Memphis City Hospital, Diggs found not only an interesting problem to satisfy his desire for research, but one with "always numerous, readily available, cooperative patients whose type of hemoglobin was already established by routine and specific tests."[35]

Medicine as a profession in Memphis, as elsewhere, was racially segregated, as were all public and private institutions in the city. The only black workers in the hospital were maintenance and janitorial workers. Vivien Thomas, a black laboratory technician aspiring to be a doctor, was the exception that proved the rule. He began his career at Vanderbilt University in Nashville and moved during the Great Depression to Baltimore, where he began a lifelong collaboration with Alfred Blalock, the same surgeon who treated Diggs's concussion.[36] As one historian points out, the number of white medical schools in 1900 numbered 160 and the number of black schools numbered 10. By 1930 there were 76 white schools and 2 black ones. The educational transformation that began with the Flexner Report resulted in a more homogeneous, that is to say white, medical profession.[37] In Memphis the private hospitals were affiliated with religious organizations.

Diggs took stock of the patients in the Memphis City Hospital. Within the first few days he became interested in the high number of sickle cell patients that he observed. He thought back to his days as a resident at the University of Rochester where he had administered liver extract to patients with thalassemia, a disease similar to sickle cell. Thalassemia is also found in people from the Mediterranean, Africa, and Asia. He had been taught that sickle cell was a rare disease, yet here on his wards it seemed relatively common. He had received vials of liver extract from Dr. Whipple before leaving Rochester: "Dr. Whipple gave me some samples of liver extract to test out on people with iron deficiency anemia and pellagra which was then present."[38] On the speculative assumption that sickle cell might be metabolic or nutritional in nature, Diggs gave the extract to some of his patients without effect. Nevertheless, his interest in sickle cell was piqued and would be sustained throughout his career.

George Whipple had asked Diggs to use the ampules of liver extract on patients with iron deficiency anemia or pellagra but, on the assumption that sickle cell might be metabolic or nutritional, Diggs's thought was to give the liver extract to his sickle cell patients, which he knew had not been tried elsewhere, along with other anti-anemic drugs. He tried this approach for several years, with disappointing results. The solution to the disease did not appear to lie in nutrition. He also considered giving the extract to the patients with pellagra, a disease with similar symptoms. But something about sickle cell interested and even intrigued him. Perhaps because the disease was both little understood and appropriate for the use of the technology that was close to him—the microscope and the clinical laboratory—sickle cell inspired his abiding commitment. It was one of the few diseases at the time that could be diagnosed microscopically. This could not be said of diseases such as pellagra, for which others were studying the therapeutic benefit of liver extract.[39]

The Memphis City Hospital also included the Pathology Institute, where Diggs did much of his work and teaching. Pathology as a subspecialty was seen as an important source of new medical knowledge. It was highly regarded because doctors could only hypothesize about what was going on inside a body while a patient was alive, and there was no way to look inside short of surgery. X-rays were helpful in imaging the inside a body, but only insofar as the images represented tissue densities. Soft tissues were very hard to read and often fell far short of providing useful information. And radiology was still evolving as a clinical tool. Thus case reports were frequently published with autopsy results.

O. W. Hyman, the UT Medical Units' chief administrator, viewed Pathology as a key department. He was cognizant of the growing need for such a department as a training program, as a basic science, and as a service, and he wanted to create a first-rate pathology program for the university. To that end, he hired Harry Christian Schmeisser, also trained at Hopkins, from Emory University in 1921 and asked him to reorganize the department. Hyman wrote that Schmeisser "brought to Memphis a clear concept of what should be done to develop a first-class Department of Pathology and Bacteriology, and during the next several years was able to supplement the staff and rearrange the work so that by the time he had been in Memphis five years, the University had a good Department of Pathology."[40] By 1929, a new crop of faculty members had replaced those of 1921. This group included Israel D. Michelson, trained at Hopkins, who was an associate professor by 1929, and Anna Dean Dulaney, with a medical degree in bacteriology from the University of Missouri, who was an assistant professor. In addition, there were also two instructors.[41]

Although pathology was respected as a basic medical science, the use of laboratory tests as a functional part of clinical medicine was controversial in Memphis, as elsewhere. "Laboratory tests," as Diggs noted, "were not at first universally accepted. It was felt by some that reliance upon the laboratory for diagnosis would encourage laziness on the part of the clinician and abandonment of established practice."[42] This feeling was generally accepted by many of the older and senior-level physicians in Memphis. The worry was that physicians, who came to rely on laboratory testing for information about their patients, would lose the vital skill to exercise their clinical judgment based on the use of their five senses to understand and treat their patients. For many, the ideal doctor was the one who could operate a solo practice and make all the important assessments without waiting for a nurse or a technician. As late as 1924, one local physician wrote, "A physician who cannot prescribe for the average patient or who will not venture a diagnosis until after he shall have had submitted to him the reports of internes and nurses, with their interpretations of the findings of the various specimens submitted, will never be able to take care of the sick and injured of an isolated community."[43] This attitude was a barrier for Diggs and others, who were establishing the clinical laboratory as an essential resource for patient care.

Furthermore, behind this concern, there was a growing statewide need for physicians in rural areas of Tennessee. Doctors who specialized or who required laboratory tests and personnel were more likely to practice in the cities, rather than in the midsize or smaller towns where the need for healthcare was deemed urgent. To be sure, laboratories were considered important, but they would never replace the clinical judgment of a trained physician. As one of the new generation of doctors, Diggs represented those who embraced the new view, who did not question the value of the laboratory, and who sought to find ways to expand its use in clinical medicine. In an extension of his experience at the University of Rochester, he applied all the laboratory techniques he could to helping his patients. From the beginning as a part of the medical school curriculum, Diggs taught a course in clinical pathology as well as exercising his responsibility as the coordinator of the laboratory that was part of the Pathology Institute. In this he had the support of his department chair.

There was one black-owned hospital with a small number of beds, the Collins Chapel Hospital, that opened in 1910. The Memphis City Hospital, including its cafeteria, was segregated, yet it was the only one that African Americans could use, since all the other hospitals in the city were private and white. The patient population did not reflect the city population, which was 38.1 percent black; many of these people represented the early twentieth-century mass migration from rural communities to the cities. The percentage of blacks in the hospital was about 80, because it was the only hospital to which they would have been admitted. The building had a central three-story administrative and central services tower with two, two-story, arms of patients' rooms extending at an angle from either side. The tower had a dome that was modeled after the well-known one atop Johns Hopkins's hospital in Baltimore, a sign of the influence that the famous medical school had exerted, and a tacit reflection of the Flexner Report, which had used the Johns Hopkins School of Medicine as a measure for evaluating all of the medical schools in the country.[44]

By 1929 the Memphis City Hospital had transitioned from the almshouse and charity model of the nineteenth century to one that aligned itself with the cascade of medical innovations and the science that produced them. By this time it was a place where health could be restored, instead of a place where the chronically ill went to die. The hospital had adopted a business model and was attempting to attract middle-class patients. "Dumping," the practice of transferring extremely ill or seriously injured accident victims from one hospital to another, also began at about this time in an effort to avoid expensive illnesses or to improve hospital death rates. No independent or federal regulations for hospitals or doctors existed at this time.[45]

The sickle cell patients whom Diggs saw had a recognizable syndrome, a set of symptoms including a jaundiced appearance, skin ulcers (usually on the legs), painful abdominal and joint crises, and the familiar abnormally shaped red blood cells. From the point of view of the patients, the hallmark of this illness was the excruciating pain "out of the clear sky oftentimes," as Diggs described:

> And, the pains are in multiple parts of the body, but usually they are in the back or in the bones. As they say, "It bees bones." And, they put their hands on the bones. But, this pain is very severe and it makes them scream and cry and they, it's like an abscessed tooth or a kidney stone or gallstone colic. It's very severe pain and it makes them seek medical aid and go to the emergency room and to go to the hospital. And, it's the type of thing that occurs over again and really is a curse of the people who have sickle cell anemia and that is one of the efforts in research, is to try to find out how to prevent these crises and how to treat them after they occur.[46]

These symptoms appeared in a variety of places, which gave rise to a number of possible causes, but none of them could account for all of the symptoms together. Thus, misdiagnosis of the disease was frequent. The ability of sickle cell to mimic other diseases led Maxwell Wintrobe to label it a "little imitator" as early as 1937. Ten years later another writer would call it a "great masquerader" in the tradition of William Osler's reference to syphilis and tuberculosis.[47] In time it would be recognized that sickle cell could be mistaken for appendicitis, perforated ulcer, tuberculosis peritonitis, rheumatic fever, osteomyelitis, syphilis, pneumonia, encephalitis, arthritis, rheumatic heart disease, meningitis, malaria, cerebral embolism, and a variety of diseases producing anemia or jaundice.[48] There was nothing that Diggs could do for the patient apart from trying to treat the symptoms. No way had been identified conceptually to link the manifestations of sickle cell anemia to an underlying cause. Moreover, the accumulation of clinical statistics would not be useful in forming a picture of the disease for the same reason. As a young physician beginning his career and establishing his reputation, Diggs saw an opportunity that intrigued him and superbly fit his professional training and inclinations.

If the clinical findings from his patients were unhelpful, so was the medical literature. "There was no one had any interest in it," he recalled.[49] One of the first things he did was to find out how much had been published on sickle cell that could augment what he knew. In keeping with his scientific training and habit, he sought to assemble everything that was known about the disease at that time. Diggs noted, "In 1929 the description of clinical, laboratory, and anatomical manifestations related to sickle cell anemia in the major textbooks were [sic] limited to a few lines, and there were few indexed publications."[50] To this end, he spent time reading what there was in medical journals and prominent textbooks. He scanned the English textbooks that he could identify, underlining what he thought important.[51] In addition, he studied various German textbooks. Many of the words on the page were cognates, and thus recognizable as medical terms. With a German-English dictionary nearby, Diggs translated the meanings of the non-medical words onto the book page in order to decipher the meaning of the text.[52] The textbooks in general contained very little useful information.

More important than the textbook information, however, was what could be found in the medical literature. All new ideas, conjectures, and clinically and scientifically significant findings were published in the pages of journals that served not only as the first exposure for new and novel ideas but also as the means of communication between researchers. Diggs wanted to know everything there was on the disease from the time it had first been described in 1910. He thumbed through copies of *Quarterly Cumulative Index Medicus*, the specialized subject-heading and author catalog of all medical journal publications, searching for relevant citations.[53] The results were meager. Information about the disease was both limited and confusing. He acquired copies of all the relevant articles that had been published to that time by using the interlibrary loan services of the newly built C. P. J. Mooney Library located across the street from his office and named after the editor-in-chief of the Memphis newspaper *The Commercial Appeal.* He requested reprints from article authors by mail (a standard practice at the time), requested photo duplications of articles on interlibrary loan, and sometimes used a typewriter to reproduce an article. Diggs followed the same research instinct that he would use throughout his career. He not only read the articles to supplement his own knowledge about sickle cell and other diseases, but also began a filing system of those articles to keep them organized for himself and for others interested in the disease, a habit that would grow over the next four decades from a filing system into an essential, inclusive research resource; Diggs and others in Memphis would come to refer to these materials as a knowledge base of what was understood about the disease and as a source of ideas for future research.[54] The indexed articles were contained occasional marginal comments in Diggs's hand in the form of corrections or updates to an author's assertions. In one instance, an author asserted, "The true sickle cells in the blood of an active case are absolutely unaffected by oxygen." To this, Diggs wrote a firm "NO!" in the margin.[55]

Diggs relied on the contents of the literature to guide his work and to help him understand the clinical, laboratory, anatomical, and pathological manifestations of sickle cell anemia. He would routinely refer in his own publications to the number of journal articles available on the subject and would include either a complete list of those articles or at least the significant ones. His purpose was not only the practical purpose of showing where he had obtained his information, but simply to begin with what was already known.

Diggs supplemented what he had learned as John Huck's student at Hopkins, where he saw and heard about sickle cell anemia for the first time. He knew that the disease had first been described in 1910 by James B. Herrick, whose patient had leg ulcers, yellow sclera (jaundice), anemia, and the peculiar "thin, elongated, sickle-shaped" red blood cells that would characterize the disease. Herrick could not diagnose the cause or do anything more than suggest that it was possibly the result of syphilis or an intestinal parasite.[56] A similar case was described a year later.[57] In 1915 Jerome Cook and Jerome Meyer reported a third, similar case, in which the authors stated for the first time that the symptoms defined a new disease that was probably limited to blacks. On the basis of the three known cases, they started a trend toward identifying the inherited nature of the disease that would become a central element in the definition of sickle cell.[58] At about the same time, Victor Emmel developed a laboratory test that could demonstrate the sickling of red cells in symptomatic and some asymptomatic people. With this technology, he used a blood sample from the non-anemic father of Cook and Meyer's patient—someone who had never manifested the symptoms of the disease—to show that his red cells would sickle on a glass slide under a microscope, thus demonstrating that someone without the disease could manifest a "trait" for the disease. This meant that something of the disease that the patient had was also found in the patient's father, which indicated that the disease was familial in nature. With this test, Emmel moved the discussion away from the clinical assessment of symptoms to the cellular nature of the disease, and to discussion of an active disease with a trait that could also be found in otherwise normal individuals.[59]

John Huck, Diggs's teacher at Hopkins, performed the first comprehensive studies of sickling that resulted in a definition of a dominant trait according to the Mendelian laws of inheritance for a single factor. Only one parent with the dominant trait was required to transmit the disease to the child. Henceforth, sickle cell would be cast as an inheritable disease. Huck also made no distinction between those individuals possessing the trait and those with the active disease: the phenomenon of sickling was considered an indication of the disease, and the disease could be found on a spectrum from severe to absent, which led to the odd notion that a person could be healthy and have a disease, both at the same time.[60] This conclusion was due in part to the lack of any test that could distinguish between those with the disease and those with the trait who would never manifest the disease. Emmel claimed that his test alone could be used for drawing inferences about the disease, in contrast to the earlier practice of grouping patients as the means for defining the disease. In 1922 another researcher, Verne Mason, would echo the importance of the laboratory findings, but stressed the need to include the clinical manifestations in any diagnosis, something that Diggs later underscored.[61]

Virgil P. Sydenstricker added his observations to the handful that had been made before him. In 1923 he examined two patients (two and six years of age) suffering from the disease and their families, using Emmel's test for "latent" sickling. The younger patient died. However, probably for the first time, Sydenstricker used the opportunity to examine the body to see the effects that the disease had had on the child, noting changes to the spleen, kidneys, and bone marrow. He made an early reference to the possibility that the problem might be the hemoglobin of the red cells: "The cells became darker and more 'brassy' as though there were a concentration of the hemoglobin."[62] The suspicion of hemoglobin as the center of the problem would remain elusive until after World War II. Sydenstricker also added his weight to the speculation that "sickle cell anemia is a condition peculiar to the negro race."[63]

Sydenstricker held that the condition of the blood and the hereditary nature of the disease were crucial for diagnosis, while maintaining a central concern for the clinical picture.[64] As Feldman and Tauber explained, "Sydenstricker's analysis entailed that a patient's diagnosis may change over time as the phase of the disease changes. Thus, while he drew no etiological boundary between phases, he believed in an underlying structural reason for the differences. He introduced the term 'crisis' in his 1924 paper on sickle cell anemia to describe the acute and painful manifestations of sickle cell anemia in its active phase, which he saw as a cyclical pattern of remission and relapse." His observations would lay the groundwork for much of the later research on sickle cell anemia.[65]

The first case of sickle cell in Memphis was reported in 1925 by J. F. Hamilton to the Memphis and Shelby County Medical Society, with the clinical aspects of a local thirty-three-year-old black farmer and World War

I veteran, who was seen by Hamilton in U.S. Veterans Hospital No. 88 with the familiar complaints of abdominal and joint pain, leg ulcers, a jaundiced appearance, and the characteristic sickle-shaped red cells. The main purpose of Hamilton's report, apart from the significance of this being the first case, was to briefly review the literature and to note that the disease appeared "to occur only in the colored race," that it was a rare disease, and that it was transmitted by the laws of Mendelian inheritance.[66] At least one other case was reported in 1927, at the Memphis City Hospital, just two years before Diggs arrived. The so-called rarity of the disease underscored Diggs's surprise at finding a higher number of cases than he expected.[67]

As poorly understood as Diggs found the disease to be among physicians, blacks were almost completely unaware that it existed, although the phenomenon was well known and often signaled by the painful cries of its sufferers.[68] The fatigue caused by the anemia was often identified as "malingering," the joint pain as "rheumatism" or "arthritis," and the other symptoms as "other diseases," including malaria. Financial support for blacks in the form of health insurance was virtually unknown, which meant that sufferers would not go to the hospital until the illness was unbearable and usually quite advanced; under such conditions, they were also less likely to pay after they had left the hospital. In segregated hospitals, a black patient had the most difficult time being admitted, but if that hurdle could be overcome, the quality of care was only marginally worse than for white patients. Prejudices among the hospital staff did not disappear, but were usually made secondary to professional standards. Most hospital staff members would extend themselves to provide the same quality of care to blacks as to whites, but only as long as the patients were compliant to the staff's orders. If a black patient resisted care or refused to obey, racial prejudices would emerge and could be harsh. As one physician at a Houston charity hospital put it, "we are forced to treat the poor Negroes as another species, test animals, relics of the Stone Age not as sensitive as we to pain."[69]

Diggs never charged his sickle cell patients a fee.[70] This was a help to his patients, but also served to encourage them to return to him, thus providing a small but growing group of patients that he could follow and learn from. Charity existed as an ideal shared by physicians, in which doctor-patient relations were central and the doctor would offer to treat those who could not pay. This image continued to be central to the American Medical Association as part of the ideal of the doctor as a professional.[71]

Hospitals also reflected that ideal, but in practicality could not afford it, for even though the doctor might not charge a fee for services, the services of the hospital, including nursing, equipment, and laboratory supplies, did have a cost attached to them that was lost when the patient did not pay. Private hospitals especially would reduce as far as possible the number of nonpaying patients that they received, whereas public hospitals often could not refuse to treat anyone who came through their doors.

The perspective of white physicians was often less than charitable toward blacks. A Texas physician wrote in 1916, "It must be evident, therefore, that the negro race is responsible not only for its own high rate of mortality, but must also bear some burden of responsibility for the dissemination of disease and death among the whites."[72] Because of the reported population distribution, the author asserted that the poor health of blacks was essentially a southern problem, one that for whites was "greatly intensified by our negro population." He went on to say, "When we remember that the negroes of the South, our servants in intimate association with our families from the cradle to the grave, are widely infected, we can begin to understand how innocent infections may be widespread."[73] The author concluded that the magnitude of the problem that the black population posed for the white population was as yet not fully appreciated, and called for additional efforts to define the problem more precisely.

Closer to home, the Memphis Superintendent of Health, L. M. Graves, reported in 1929 to the Shelby County Medical Society on the public health of the city. Rather than present a comprehensive picture, he focused on the five top troublesome illnesses of the day: typhoid, malaria, tuberculosis, diphtheria, and scarlet fever. Tuberculosis and typhoid were of greatest concern because of their high incidence and high death rates, which he attributed both to nonresidents and to Memphis blacks. The reference to the nonresident population was due in part to the fact that Memphis had the only big-city hospital for over a hundred-mile radius, and to the demographic pattern of migration from the countryside to the cities.[74] The situation regarding tuberculosis caused one doctor to state, "the negro is the most important factor that we should place under control, if we ever hope to control tuberculosis"; another doctor agreed that "our plan of attack, especially in a population such as we have in Memphis, must give more consideration to the colored element."[75]

Among Diggs's main duties in his new position was to teach clinical pathology and to supervise the clinical laboratories of the Memphis City Hospital. He was considered a thorough instructor, the kind who was so well organized in his lectures that students could readily take good class notes.[76] The patients of this city hospital were generally those who were sick and poor. There was one wing for whites and another for blacks, but at any given time, most of the patients in the hospital, around 80 percent were black. These patients suffered from the wide range of diseases seen in public hospitals at the time. Sickle cell anemia was still poorly understood, despite having first been described in 1910 (almost twenty years earlier), and it was considered rare. No one had any idea of the prevalence of the disease. Diggs had learned how to identify it microscopically in medical school, and was struck by the number of patients he now saw in Memphis; he wondered what he could learn that would help those suffering from the illness.

For the first few years at the University of Tennessee Medical Units, Diggs remained intrigued by a puzzle: the disease was striking in its presentation. It could manifest itself as chronic fatigue or jaundice, and in the abdomen, joints, and elsewhere in the body, but it was always accompanied by episodes of severe and excruciating pain. At the heart of the disease were the strange abnormally shaped sickled red blood cells. As was characteristic of his research style, Diggs's first instinct was to find out everything he could about the disease.

When he was with his patients he was not a scientist, but rather a physician intent on treating their illnesses by using whatever science was available and appropriate for the treatment. He used science as a sounding board for his own ideas to help people, and if a cause could be found that would lead to an intervention, such as a drug, then his task was to reach a therapeutic and positive outcome. By contrast, in the laboratory he was a scientist involved in the activity of producing new scientific knowledge, using the discipline of a scientist together with the laboratory tools that were available.[77]

There was much to learn about the disease, and Diggs found himself immersed in sorting through the ideas presented in the literature. After his unsuccessful attempt to treat the disease as a nutritional disorder with liver extract, he began working through the puzzle more methodically. At an annual meeting of the Southern Medical Association in New Orleans in 1931, he presented his first paper on the disease, focusing on the core problem, namely, the blood picture of the disease and its diagnosis. In the 1932 publication that grew out of this presentation, Diggs criticized the common misunderstanding that sickle cell was a rare disease. In his short time at the Memphis City Hospital, he had come to understand that sickle cell was a much more common disorder than was generally recognized. The reason for this, he said, was because "the condition is unrecognized, and a knowledge of the blood picture is necessary for its recognition."[78] The disorder was not rare because the incidence was low, but rather because a greater effort was required by physicians to understand what to look for: "Although the characteristic hematological findings have been clearly stated in the past by Sydenstricker, Graham, Steinberg, and other students of the disease, there still occur in the meager treatment of the subject in recent reference books gross misstatements; and in the literature confusing terms and unwarranted generalities based upon inadequate evidence."[79] Diggs's need for clarity in language, his desire to educate others, and his emphasis on scientific rigor were evident here. Also characteristic of his science was to base the paper on a complete review of the literature and to cull sixty-four recorded cases, to which he added ten additional cases from the Memphis hospital. In this way he performed a rudimentary meta-analysis of the cases reported in the journal literature, to which he added his own data.

Diggs drew a distinction between the illness as manifested in individuals having the familiar sickled and elongated red blood cells and showing the symptoms of the disease, and as manifested in those individuals possessing the trait but who were not symptomatic. The key point for him was that far too little was known about the existence of the trait to be able to draw any meaningful conclusions. Those who possessed the trait as determined by Emmel's test without manifesting any symptoms were by definition ill. Diggs chose to bypass these people in favor of focusing on those showing symptoms. Undoubtedly those with the trait were connected to those exhibiting the disease, but Diggs chose to focus on the disease and its remedy. He argued that the latter category of individuals should be excluded from consideration for the time being because information was still confusing. He recognized that both classes represented different aspects of the same disease but were clearly distinct in that those with the disease displayed active signs, such as skin ulcers, and those with the trait (sicklemia) displayed no active signs and lived otherwise normal lives. Those individuals whose blood could be made to sickle in the laboratory by using Emmel's test, but who did not manifest the clinical features of the disease, were excluded from consideration in his first paper because too little was understood about this aspect of the disease. The essential features that Diggs discussed included sickled cells, signs of red blood cell destruction, signs of red blood cell regeneration, and a chronic and cyclical recurrence of symptoms. He argued that these four conditions had to be present for any diagnosis of sickle cell, and by definition such a diagnosis could not include those with the trait who did not have the active symptoms. Except for the ten patients that Diggs discusses, this paper was a review of the available literature and of all the cases that were reported for the common features that defined the disease, and of the statements made about the disease that were misleading and erroneous. In this latter regard, Diggs argued that, far from being rare, sickle cell was quite common. He pointed out, "countless cases of sickle cell anemia have been missed or diagnosed hemolytic jaundice, pernicious anemia or von Jaksch's anemia because these obvious sickled forms were not present."[80] It was a mistake, he was saying, to preclude sickle cell in any diagnosis of a hemolytic anemia just because the telltale misshapen red cells were absent.

Furthermore, this paper is representative of Diggs's interest in medical illustration as a means of summarizing scientific information. Joseph L. Scianni, who joined the Department of Pathology years before Diggs's arrival, was the department's artist and the illustrator of this paper. Although no one lacked admiration for the microphotograph and the immediate realism that it conveyed, it also had its limitations, such as the momentary angle of the photograph (the inability to "pose" a microscopic object) and the distortions and artifacts in the surrounding medium. The subject being shot was usually not in the ideal position or completely free of flaws. Moreover, the images were still black-and-white, so the colors seen in the microscope that were crucial to scientific understanding were absent for both the clinician and the teacher. The powerful advantage of using an artist could be seen in the undistorted and colorful image that would result; this would in turn yield valuable information for the doctor. The artist's image might be idealized, but, so the thinking went, it was often a better rendering than any microphotograph could produce, because it could contain more pertinent and better-organized visual information than in a photograph.

Of course, the artistic illustrations were only as good as the artist and knowledge that produced them, which could date an image as scientific knowledge changed. Another drawback was that the artist must be medically as well as artistically trained, and to bring the artist's medical expertise to the required level was often more expensive and more time consuming than to take a photograph with a camera. Needless to say, the camera would become widely used, because of its mechanical, objective renderings as the technology improved. Photography and x-ray images were part of a broad social movement at this time, and much effort was being made to read meaning into these new mechanical pictures; this was no less true in medicine and the sciences in general. Artists such as Scianni in the Department of Pathology; Diggs's teacher at Hopkins, Max Brödel; and others would eventually disappear.[81] Diggs could accept the neutrality and the realism of the microphotograph, but he could also acknowledge the photo's inability to capture every aspect of the subject due to randomness or the irregular symmetry of nature. The artist's rendering could ignore the imperfections and position the subject in the most advantageous way; moreover, the subject could be colored in a way that the viewer could see through the lens but that black-and-white film could not capture.

Whereas Diggs's first paper sought to define the disease based on everything that was known at that time, his second paper began to focus on the process of the disease itself. In particular, it was concerned with the rate at which red cells sickled in someone with the active disease, as contrasted with someone having the trait but not the active disease. Even as Diggs sought to establish his reputation, however, the Depression's effect on life in Memphis deepened.

Diggs's attitude towards money was acquired during his Methodist upbringing, in which money was to be earned freely and spent frugally and only on things that were necessary. He sought ways to spend money more efficiently. This was in contrast to attitudes of the 1920s, which can best be characterized as the "get-rich-quick mentality."[82] By 1932 the effects of the economic disaster had made themselves felt in full force in Memphis, and Diggs's frugal lifestyle proved most advantageous.

Diggs read widely to keep up with his areas of interest. In his perusal of the literature at the Mooney Library, he serendipitously came across an article in the *West African Medical Journal* presenting a case of malaria with a marked splenic involvement in a two-year-old boy, a type of anemia known as "von Jaksch anemia" and found in children.[83] This form of anemia would later be renamed "thalassemia."[84] E. C. Smith was a physician at the Medical Research Institute in Yaba, a suburb of Lagos, Nigeria, who reported the autopsy findings, which included a detailed description of the effects of the disease on the patient's internal organs. Diggs wrote a letter to the editor of the journal, offering his assessment of Smith's findings of "definite jaundice, fever, and marked regenerative bone marrow activity," which, he suggested, since it was found in a young Negro, also fit the syndrome of sickle cell anemia. His letter was published, and in the following month Smith responded by quoting Diggs's own findings to the journal's readers.[85] This exchange would lead to the future collaboration and exchange of information between the two doctors, especially in understanding the role of the spleen in the disease. Diggs contacted many researchers and would later claim to have been in contact and to have met everyone involved in sickle cell research at one time or another.[86]

An example of the ways in which Diggs became acquainted with other researchers was his presentation of a paper (published in 1933) on the pathology of sickle cell anemia at the Southern Medical Association Conference in Richmond. There he spoke for the first time on the likely cause of the anatomical lesions and painful crises that he and others had observed. His observations revealed the possibility that the distorted red cells were packing together and causing capillary infarction, namely blockage that prevented blood flow and resulted in tissue death in the surrounding area. "A possible explanation of the capillary engorgement is that the elongated and spiked cells interlock and pass with more difficulty through narrowed spaces than do normal cells."[87] It had already been noted that the sickling process happened in the absence of oxygen, Diggs continued, and this might account for the spontaneous appearance of painful episodes occurring anywhere in the body. Once the sickled cells formed packs, thus slowing and stopping the flow of blood, the level of oxygen in the area declined, creating a condition that prompted sickling to accelerate. Diggs gave the first indication of sickle cell anemia as an ischemic disease. This underlying mechanism of action would inform the research of Diggs and other for the next fifteen years. Research results such as these stimulated the thinking of other doctors, in turn leading to cross-fertilization of ideas and hypotheses, and moving the subject of sickle cell anemia and its treatment further toward the foreground of discussion by members of the medical-scientific community.

The impact of this capillary packing of red cells led to an unfortunate but instructive incident involving the surgical removal of a spleen as a last resort to help a young woman with sickle cell symptoms that began early in life and had persisted: "At school and while working in the cotton fields, the patient tired more easily than other children and took little part in their play."[88] Every therapy was tried to alleviate the young woman's condition, but to no avail. Diggs noted that she had what he thought was an enlarged spleen. As a last resort, Diggs considered allowing the surgical removal of her spleen. Sickle cell patients with enlarged spleens were thought to be anemic, in part because of the sickling of the red cells, which were removed by the body's immune system, and also by a malfunctioning spleen, which many thought withdrew and eliminated normal red cells. According to Mabry and Diggs, "People who had severe anemia and had jaundice associated with anemia and other diseases, hereditary spherocytosis (red cells that are spherical instead of biconcave), were profited sometimes if you removed this big spleen which was a destroyer of red cells, and you could help to restore their balance and make them less anemic."[89]

The chief of surgery, Lucius McGehee, performed the surgery with assistance from the chief of medicine, J. E. McElroy. Because of the historic nature of the operation, it was performed in the surgical amphitheater with the senior medical students invited to observe. After opening the abdomen, Dr. McGehee was unable to find the spleen. What had appeared to be a large spleen on physical examination turned out to be an enlarged liver that had extended over into the area of the abdomen that included the spleen. "Perspiration broke out over his forehead, and his brow was repeatedly wiped by the operating room nurses. He enlarged the incision, resected a rib, and shifted his retractors to get better visualization," all to no avail. In frustration, McGehee was heard to mutter that he would eat the spleen, which normally weighs 150 to 200 grams, if it weighed 10 grams. The chief of medicine could not resist a joke at the expense of the hapless surgeon by pointing out that "we would do better if we had more competent surgeons."[90]

Despite every effort, the young woman died the following day; after her death an autopsy was performed. Hoping to salvage something from the previous day's embarrassment, Dr. McGehee attended the autopsy to continue his search. This time he was rewarded with success. The spleen was found adhering to the diaphragm, small and almost unrecognizable. It weighed 7.5 grams. Thus, Dr. McGehee did not have to eat it, but it raised an important question in Diggs's mind: how could an organ shrink to almost nothing on its own? Diggs published the negative findings of this surgery along with a review of the literature on similar splenectomies, in which he argued against removing the spleen until much more was learned about its role in the disease.[91] "If left alone, they will in effect 'splenectomize' themselves without the benefit of surgery."[92] His interest in and growing knowledge about this mysterious disease were deepening.

This surgical experience was reported in the *Archives of Internal Medicine* and was followed by articles about other instances of spleens that seemed to just disappear. Diggs was thus motivated to try to work out "what the sequence of events [was] in the spleen that first was large and later became small."[93] There was another case in which the spleen shrank to a size that made it impossible to find: "We traced the place where it ought to be and made sections of a little scar tissue where it ought to be and it wasn't there."[94] The experience of seeing an entire organ disappear spurred on Diggs's interest in this disease. "I tried to know why in the world that spleen had disappeared or had gotten so small."[95] He understood that infarctions were caused by the bizarre shapes of red cells, together with the cells' sensitivity to low oxygen levels, but if this could happen to the spleen, what could be occurring in any of the other organs in the body? "In other words, the spleen can actually disappear in these people on account of the fact that the sickled cells plug up the capillaries and the spleen just doesn't have blood supply and it just atrophies and goes away."[96] Starting from this point, Diggs's focus was on the effect that the disease had on organ systems, and this focus would continue for the remainder of his career.

In these years from 1929 to the 1940s, Diggs did not have a relationship with the African American community. He was preoccupied with learning his responsibilities as a faculty member, teacher, clinician, and laboratory supervisor. As an assistant professor, his duties were limited to conducting research and publishing in the medical journals, teaching, seeing patients, and serving on campus committees and in professional organizations. Diggs chose to do active research in conjunction with his clinical duties even though it was expected but not encouraged; he did not have a quota of publications to meet, and did not necessarily have to publish in the major medical journals. Promotion in rank was often treated as a perfunctory activity and usually at the discretion of the department chair. Faculty members were sometimes informed of their promotion without the knowledge that they were even being considered for promotion.

After the clinical and research work, the bulk of Diggs's time was spent on teaching. In 1930 the campus changed its curriculum from a two-semester to a four-quarter program. A four-quarter program had been discussed for several years at a number of medical schools. The chief business officer, O. W. Hyman, adopted a plan that incorporated the maximum flexibility for students, which was achieved by offering all of the courses in the medicine curriculum in every quarter. The advantage for students was that they could complete their degrees in as little as three and one-quarter years. In addition, if they needed to earn money for tuition or living expenses, students could opt out at the end of any quarter and resume their studies one or two quarters later without having to repeat any courses or risking the loss of any academic standing. The clear disadvantage to the faculty was that the new system increased teaching loads by requiring them to teach all courses every semester.[93] Such an increase in the workload for faculty was burdensome and came at a time when the Tennessee budget would not allow the hiring of additional faculty.

Just as the Great Depression exposed the weaknesses of the American economic system, it starkly exposed the weaknesses of the healthcare system. If the loss of capital and unemployment was bad, it was in all aspects worse for African Americans because they had access to fewer resources and were assigned a lower social position. Blacks were uninformed about sickle cell anemia but were undoubtedly familiar with symptoms they could not understand, and they had no means to find doctors who would treat their symptoms. The symptoms were debilitating and recurring, which meant a considerable expense for the sufferers. Hospital stays ranged from several days to several weeks and, by 1917, hospitals in Memphis were already charging all patients two dollars for routine blood and urinalysis tests.[94] For someone earning very little, it would be easy for a visit to the doctor or hospital to amount to a week's or a month's income.

In order for Diggs to study sickle cell in his patients, he needed to have systematic access to them. It was not enough to see patients as they appeared in the hospital; he would need to follow them over time. This was a daunting task, considering that his patients were often unable to come to the hospital, either because they did not understand the nature of their illness or, just as often, because they could not afford to pay the fees that would be required. There was no research funding for a disease that no one considered important. The disease was expensive for families because of the recurring, painful crises (estimated at four to six per year on average) that required the attention of a physician, and often the crises were so severe that they required admission to a hospital for several days or weeks. "Transportation, laboratory tests, medicines, and sometimes the cost of intravenous solutions and/or transfusions" added to the cost of the disease. As Diggs and Ernestine T. Flowers observed, "Any single crisis requiring intravenous therapy may cost more than the total weekly earnings of the family."[95]

Although irregular, these crises could occur as often as four to six times per year. Surgical supplies and complications, such as gallstones, blood in the urine, osteomyelitis, pulmonary emboli, and so on, could also add to the medical expense. Moreover, absence from school and inability to participate in childhood activities interfered with the education and training of the sufferers, and could lead to an inferiority complex. In general, sickle cell patients were handicapped and needed to plan their lives accordingly. They needed to have a job that allowed them to contribute to their support, but not jobs with sustained physical exertion, such as heavy lifting, or exposure to extreme heat, cold, dehydration, or low oxygen levels. Sickle cell posed a challenge for employers because recurrent illnesses caused the afflicted to miss too much time from their work; hence jobs that did not require daily, uninterrupted attendance were ideal. Given the challenges facing the people with the disease and doctors seeking to learn more about it, Diggs quickly realized that part of the solution for coping with this disease lay in the education of everyone involved, including patients, families, healthcare personnel, teachers, social and welfare case workers, rehabilitation and job-training counselors, and insurance companies.[96]

There was genuine suspicion in the black community about doctors who might experiment on patients out of an overzealous sense of scientific curiosity; this sentiment was deeply seated and widespread. For a physician such as Diggs, who was seeking the participation of his patients in scientific studies, the task was one of convincing them that his motives and procedures were the highest and noblest. At this time in American medicine, the profession expected that patients be asked for their consent before participating in any kind of study, although it was less clear to what extent they should be fully informed of the consequences of the study. In general, consent was left to the discretion of the physician.[97]

Despite the high regard that medicine enjoyed and in the absence of any codified policy of informed consent in any kind of investigation, there were lingering fears in society in general about medicine's "true" aims. Prisoners, orphaned children, and those deemed "idiots" were involved in scientific experiments in the absence of any formal guidelines and without their full knowledge of the risks they were taking. An organized response to these concerns was the antivivisectionist movement, which began in the last quarter of the nineteenth century and lasted through the twentieth century. It raised compelling issues concerning who should be allowed to participate in medical research and under what circumstances. As Susan E. Lederer noted, "For the antivivisectionists, exploitation was the issue."[98] This public concern must have played a role in the minds of Diggs's patients. At the same time, physicians felt the criticism as an attack on the science they were so closely allied with and the very integrity of their charge to help those afflicted. One prominent Memphis physician reacted this way to groups opposing experimentation: "One of these is a society whose influence is felt even in the American Congress called Antivivisectionists whose sole purpose seems to be to block the way at the very threshold of scientific research and who regard the lives of beasts and birds or the bodies of the dead as being more sacred than the lives and health of human beings. For without a knowledge of anatomy there could be no knowledge of disease, without experimental therapeutics no knowledge of cures and without vivisection no advance in surgical procedures."[99]

Arguments on both sides were passionate and persistent. Diggs would have to work very hard to overcome public attitudes and the "Jim Crow" prejudice of the day to assure his patients that his work was in their best interest and would not harm them.[100] He had the achievements of medicine on his side. Clinical medicine was well established by the 1920s and 1930s as evidenced by the discovery of insulin, sulfa drugs, and the new treatments for pernicious anemia that were part of the small but growing cascade of innovations trumpeted in the public media. He would have to take pains to ensure that he secured the consent of those who would work with him at a time when there were no formal guidelines to direct him or any physician concerning how his work was to be done.

Sickle cell anemia was reasonably well defined by the symptoms that distinguished it from every other disease. The pieces of the puzzle were there, but what was lacking was a convincing way of explaining how the pieces fit together. The most striking piece, the sickle-shaped red cells, served only as a marker for the disease, but shed little therapeutic light. There existed no understanding of how or why the cells became deformed in this way, and no way to explain *how* or even *if* these deformities contributed to the illness. In broad terms, Diggs was trying to advance his understanding of a crippling disease during a decade, the 1930s, that was concerned with the anatomical development of the disease, its natural history, and the ways these changes manifested themselves physically in the signs and symptoms the patient or doctor might recognize.

As Diggs became more knowledgeable about sickle cell anemia, and with his wife becoming acclimated to the campus, the city, and the university, it became clear to him that understanding the disease would require more than just medical knowledge. He would also have to understand the individual and social contexts of the disease, which would require long-term follow-up visits with his patients to monitor the manifestations and natural history of the disease. As he established himself at the university and in the community, he would have to find ways to broaden his investigation, as well as educate his colleagues. At the same time, there were new ideas in the air that he would be called upon to implement, such as the recent opening of a new blood bank at Cook County Hospital in Chicago, which he would duplicate in Memphis. Diggs was thirty-eight, and about to enter his peak years.

Ah, but a man's reach should exceed his grasp,
Or what's a heaven for?
—Robert Browning, *Andrea del Sarto*

Chapter 3

Laboratory Medicine and Blood Transfusion

Diggs worked through most of his first decade with the University of Tennessee to establish himself as a faculty member and to build his reputation as a physician. He was known for his interest in sickle cell anemia. In publications and conferences, he had focused on what was known about the disease, how it was clinically defined, and the indications for further study in order to find a cure. He knew most, if not all, of the sickle cell researchers in the world, and communicated with them regularly. He was well aware that sickle cell carried a stigma, which made it difficult for his colleagues in Memphis and elsewhere to appreciate what he was doing. But if sickle cell was an "invisible" disease to all but a few in the medical research community, changes in blood banking and transfusion were about to put it in the public light.

Diggs's professional work included other diseases of the blood, such as leukemia, blood coagulation, blood group compatibility diseases, bone marrow diseases, and bleeding disorders. Because of his active involvement in the treatment of these diseases, his reputation was growing. In 1937 he provided a local lawyer, W. E. Quick, with a medical opinion in the case of a twelve-year-old girl who had been injured in a playground accident and subsequently diagnosed with chronic myeloid leukemia, "in which the marrow or myeloid cells of the body are involved." The lawyer's concern was whether the trauma of the playground accident caused the disease, to which Diggs responded in a five-page, single-spaced letter that it could not have caused the disease. Using his instincts as an educator, he instructed the lawyer on the natural history of the disease and laid out all the essential details before giving his professional opinion.[1]

As his reputation was growing, so was his family. Beatrice gave birth to their first son, Walter, in 1932. Two years later, Alice was born, and after two more years they produced another son, John. During the Depression, salaries were reduced and then remained flat for many years. Diggs felt the need for added income to support the needs of his family. He wanted to build an environment that included a home with enough land for a garden and outdoor activities. He had worked in his family's garden as a boy in Hampton, Virginia, but in the economically depressed 1930s a garden offered the added benefit of providing inexpensive food for his family. Over the years, the garden would be a fixture of the Diggs household that he would often refer to as his "country club."[2] By 1933, purchased his first home, on Evergreen Street.

Just as the Diggs family was changing, so was the environment at the University of Tennessee Medical Units. After seventy years of service to the Memphis community, the city slated a new building to replace the Memphis City Hospital about a block away on Madison Avenue. Teresa Gaston, the wife of a well-known Memphis businessman, donated part of the money for the new building. When she died, she stipulated that a part of her inheritance should be used to build a new city charity hospital to be named after her husband, John. Plans were begun as early as 1934, but, although sizeable, the amount of the inheritance was not enough to meet the projected cost of the new building. Local and state agencies were without resources because their revenue sources, such as property taxes, had declined. Like many local and state governments, Memphis turned a wary eye to Washington for support. As Roger Biles explained, Memphis "valued the federal largess, but not the ideological underpinnings of the New Deal. Memphians gratefully allowed the alphabet agencies to pick up the tab for work relief—as long as no strings came attached."[3] In the absence of any strings, the Memphis city government took advantage of the help from the federal government through the Public Works Administration, one of the many new programs started by Franklin Roosevelt's administration to assist in major building initiatives, which awarded $8,494,048 for a variety of construction projects, including the new hospital. With the help of the WPA, the John Gaston Hospital opened its doors to the public in 1936.[4]

For Diggs, the new hospital offered welcome, if short-lived, advantages in patient care. He noted that, unlike the old city hospital with its more centralized laboratory facilities, "small subsidiary laboratories were installed [in the new Gaston Hospital] as functioning units of each ward with the idea that laboratory procedures could be rapidly performed in convenient locations."[5] The benefit to patients and students was obvious to Diggs, because he evaluated hospital settings by the efficacy of patient care, which meant easy access of the doctors and technologists to clinical laboratories. These subsidiary laboratories on each ward also offered a teaching advantage by making it quick and easy for students to perform standard and simple tests for immediate results. However, the city categorized functions performed by students as "teaching," and as such considered that the cost of the subsidiary laboratories should be borne by the university. But the university was unable to afford this cost. At the same time, students objected to performing tests on patients that were not their own.

Despite Diggs's support of the educational and patient-care advantages of subsidiary laboratories, all of them were eliminated except for two. As Diggs noted, "In these laboratories, physicians in training still have the opportunity to see and to learn about the value of immediate answers to immediate problems, and the information that can be gained by simple chemical and microscopic procedures."[6] This struggle over city and state responsibility for expenditures would manifest itself in other ways over the years, but Diggs felt the loss of these basic laboratories as a setback for the hospital and its patients. The perceived low value of clinical laboratories made them an easy target for cost cutting, but their removal was also a reminder of the tension that existed between traditionally minded physicians who rejected testing as a weakening of a physician's judgment and the new generation of physicians for whom laboratory testing was an indispensible part of patient care and clinical research: "Ultimately all of the subsidiary laboratories were closed with the exception of a laboratory in the Emergency Unit and the 'Medical Student Laboratory' in the Department of Medicine."[7] Along with the setback, Diggs felt a growing frustration at the slow pace of change.

Faculty salaries remained flat during the Depression, a result of the effort by O. W. Hyman, the campus's business manager and dean of the College of Medicine, to run the campus as economically as possible. As part of his contract with the medical school, Diggs was allowed to see a limited number of private patients, although he did not have a private practice as such. His salary was based on his teaching hours, but private patients were allowed to supplement his income, which was further restricted by his choice of patients, many of whom could not pay him. He would visit his patients on the way to work or on the way home. There were so many that the time it took him to see them caused the administration to ask him to reduce the number. The administrative request was one of a growing number of frustrations. He wanted to see his income increase in recognition of his contributions to the profession and the university.

Diggs had never been interested primarily in making money. He wanted to be a hematologist, and he liked being a skeptic, but he needed the funds for his growing family. He could have gone into private practice, or chosen a more lucrative disease to investigate than sickle cell, or selected wealthier patients for his limited private practice. The situation on the University of Tennessee campus was not dire, but the Depression may have tested the will of the state legislature to continue to support this expensive and relatively new branch of the university system. The faculty was composed largely of volunteers with only a handful of full-time professors, Diggs among them. Many faculty physicians graduated from the same program and were grateful to have jobs in an ideal profession, for many among the first in their families. The work hours were long, and the money was short.

During the Depression years, many faculty members were satisfied just to have jobs. Nevertheless, the medical curriculum was heavily weighted toward education, with little or no support or encouragement for research. At least part of the burden for Diggs and the faculty in general was the academic structure adopted for the campus in 1930, known as the four-quarter plan. As Diggs knew, the idea for the plan grew out of a desire by many, mostly nonmedical colleges and universities, to take advantage of the idle summer months and make more efficient use of campus facilities. A third of the year, it was felt, was wasted because of a tradition that dated from a period when students would be called upon to work on their family farms. Since fewer and fewer students were spending their summers on the farm, or even in the countryside, the idea emerged of using this time to expand the curriculum year-round.

What made Hyman's plan for the medical school different was the requirement that all courses be taught in every quarter. The advantage for the students was plain. If they could afford to do so, they could complete the traditional four years of medical school in only three and one-quarter years. As Hyman noted, "earning periods may be alternated with study periods and the two may be varied to secure any desired sequence."[8] A number of professional athletes—football players and golfers—completed their medical degrees during the off-seasons of their sports. As an administrator, Hyman was concerned with the increasing number of physicians practicing in urban areas and, as a consequence, the aging and dwindling numbers of those remaining in small town and rural areas: "We have consciously modeled our curriculum so as to strengthen the training of graduates for practice in communities where they could not rely upon others for diagnostic aid or for help in the cure of their patients."[9] Twenty-five students were admitted per quarter, and there were four graduations each year. Tuition was kept low to make medical education affordable. Hyman understood the importance of seeking to find ways to return medical graduates to their rural Tennessee roots. Based on twenty years of data, Hyman believed that three out of four graduates would return to their small towns and rural homes to practice medicine if given an affordable medical education. As one historian noted, "the chief 'manpower' issue of American medical practice in the 1920s and 1930s was felt to be the inadequate distribution of doctors to rural areas and small communities, not the over production of specialists."[10]

Despite this admirable goal, the four-quarter plan became a disadvantage for Diggs and other faculty members because it meant more teaching hours and no prospects of hiring extra faculty to offset the increased teaching load. As a result of the increased emphasis on teaching, research and scholarly achievement were discouraged. Diggs's five-year assessment of the four-quarter plan was at odds with Hyman's conception because Diggs was convinced that research and scholarly activities were essential. The more subtle point in Diggs's reasoning was that the school was purposefully teaching physicians to diagnose and treat patients without using laboratory tests—in preparation, as Hyman put it, for a career in a small community. This flew in the face of the growing need for medical technologists. As Diggs would note: "The danger of the four-quarter system is that the advantages to the student, to the intern, to the hospital and to the state will be at the expense of the faculty, and that the advantages gained in one direction will be lost in another. Increased teaching and administrative duties, imposed by the system, unless counterbalanced by the increase in the size and caliber of the staff, will lower the standards of higher education and lead to an inferior quality of instruction."[11] The Medical Units earned a reputation for producing well-educated and capable clinicians, but little appreciation outside the region for contributions to research. Nevertheless, the four-quarter system would maintain its place through the war years and into the early 1960s. With Hyman's retirement in 1961 and the growing pressure to become more research oriented, the Medical Units soon reverted to the semester system.

Diggs was certainly pleased at the reinsertion of research in faculty life and, along with it, the growing reliance of physicians on laboratory testing. In particular, hospital physicians were increasingly incorporating laboratory tests into their patient care routines, which was felt generally as addressing a need to modernize. As early as the late 1930s, hospital physicians were ordering multiple tests on patients, often nearly every available test, whether they needed them or not. As Kenneth M. Ludmerer observed, "The level far exceeded that which was necessary for education, research, and the care of the sicker patients."[12] Hospital physicians were excessive in the tests they ordered, often with the excuse that ordering every test would cover unusual or unexpected findings. In doing so, they failed to follow their own rational and scientific approach to caring for the sick by neglecting to teach their residents and interns which laboratory tests were likely to contribute to an understanding of a patient's illness. This overuse of diagnostic tests was already beginning to contribute to the exponential increase in the cost of American medicine.[13]

Diggs also began to advocate for a program to train technicians to perform those tests as part of the medical school curriculum. He knew that the days of doctors feeling threatened by the laboratory were disappearing and were being replaced with a reliance on and expectation that laboratory testing would be available any time of the day or night. His preference was always for simple tests that could be performed even in the absence of a laboratory. This part of his thinking was consistent with Hyman's image of the community physician. But Diggs also recognized the growing number, importance, and sophistication of testing that would enhance diagnostic and therapeutic evaluations.

Although Diggs was hired initially in the Department of Pathology, he was certified in internal medicine. He believed that clinical pathology, with its patient-oriented use of laboratory techniques, represented a well-defined area within the general field of pathology. Clinical pathology used chemical analysis and other laboratory procedures for the diagnosis and treatment of disease. A professional organization, the American Association of Clinical Pathologists, was formed in 1922; Diggs felt more at home in this group than in the general field of pathology. Many of his publications in this area were contained within the pages of the journal produced by the AACP. His chair, Harry Schmeisser, could not see clinical pathology as a separate field, but rather viewed it as an indistinguishable part of pathology as the study of the nature and cause of disease based on changes in structure and function in the body.

The importance of patient care, as compared with contributing to the general knowledge of the natural history of diseases, had always motivated Diggs. In the late 1930s, he began arguing in favor of the training of technologists as a part of medical school education in order to replace the number of poorly trained technologists as quickly as possible and to alleviate the projected future need of trained technologists to perform standard tests more frequently and more efficiently than the physicians requesting them. Plus the fees hospitals charged for technologists' services represented a growing revenue stream. The days of thinking that doctors were lazy for relying on laboratory tests for their clinical work were being replaced by the belief that clinical medicine could not operate effectively or in the patient's best interest without the use of laboratory tests.[14] As a result of his difference of opinion with Schmeisser, Diggs transferred in 1937 to the Department of Medicine.[15]

One of the laboratory tests, blood matching and typing, would grow in importance for Diggs as he became interested in transfusion and blood banking. Because of its location, Memphis was vulnerable to a range of natural disasters that included thunderstorms, tornadoes, floods, and epidemics; for the people of the city, the memory lingered of the terrible yellow fever epidemics of the 1870s. At the same time, there were disasters caused by humans, such as fires, acts of violence, and various kinds of accidents. All of these events created situations in which patients would require the replacement of blood. Dramatic scenarios related to such disasters and their resulting injuries were familiar to hospitals in the 1930s, and were a part of Diggs's professional environment.

It was about this time that medical technology became a focal point for the application of scientific knowledge regarding blood-group compatibility to the problem of transfusing blood safely (as a component of patient care in medium and large city hospitals). From his readings, Diggs understood that by the mid-1930s increasing numbers of hospitals were beginning to create and staff internally operated blood banks. Russian doctors had reported success at using cadaveric blood for transfusion as early as the Crimean War in the nineteenth century, and blood banks had been reported in Spain during the Spanish Civil War.[16] It was evident that the scientific knowledge of preserving and transfusing blood had reached a point at which it could validate the creation of blood banks. The necessary supplies and testing technology were available in every hospital. As with any new innovation, the task of managing an actual blood bank meant learning about the many unforeseen problems that would arise, and taking advantage of the new opportunities that presented themselves. The time had come when the feasibility of safely storing blood for just-in-time transfusion was at hand. Diggs opened the first blood bank in the South, on the sixth floor of the John Gaston Hospital in 1938. Transfusions could begin in a matter of minutes for anyone in need of one. It is a testament both to Diggs's commitment to alleviating the suffering of patients and to the confidence the Memphis medical community placed in him that he was the doctor positioned to nurture the bank into being. Diggs was far-sighted and surely at the cutting edge of medical innovation.

Blood is culturally the most value-laden of all the body's component parts, with the possible exception of the heart. Of all the organ systems, it is the most recognizable. All people have experienced bleeding at some point in their lives, even in as simple a way as seeing their blood flow from a cut in the skin. But blood as a substance connoted much more than a red fluid of the body. Blood as a myth and symbol of life is deeply rooted in our thinking, manifesting itself in numerous ways throughout Western tradition. It participates in the language of lineage and race: "blue blood," "bloodlines," "flesh-and-blood," "bad blood," and "blood" as kinship indicate the profound sense of connections that bind people together or separate them, an ancient human feature that has endured through the centuries.[17] Given these powerful cultural associations, it should be of little wonder that the opening of a blood bank would spark a keen interest among the citizens of Memphis. What would this event mean? How would the donated blood be acquired, stored, and transfused? What guidelines would be used to determine who received it? Moreover, who would write these guidelines? People sometimes hold a lingering perception that what happens in the sciences happens in a world that operates within its own set of rules, its own methodology, and that it remains somehow separate from the extra-scientific world. Yet, as exemplified here, this is never quite the case. Technologies are never produced in apart from the society in which they originate. Diggs and other doctors witnessed the unnecessary deaths of their patients due to a lack of availability of appropriate blood that could be transfused into them quickly and safely. Their desire to save lives and advance the understanding of blood as a vital organ served as wellsprings for the creation of a blood bank.

For centuries, blood was promoted as a therapy for a range of disorders that had nothing to do with blood loss, such as lunacy, fits, palsy, melancholia, and bad disposition. In part, this practice was due to the belief that ill health was caused by bad "humors" that were poisonous, either due to imbalance or to a mysterious change in their composition. But whatever the cause, it was thought, someone with an ailment might benefit from the removal of the "bad" blood and its replacement with "good" blood, whether from a young, healthy person or an appropriate animal, such as a lamb. Physicians gave animal blood as a substitute for human blood on the assumption that some desired quality of the animal—for example, a lamb's calmness or a dog's alertness—would be transfused into the recipient.[18]

After William Harvey's hypothesis in the early seventeenth century that blood circulated in a closed system of the body, the focus by physicians turned to getting blood into and out of the body through the system of veins and arteries. Clumping was the most vexing problem. Once motionless, blood began to form clumps, which interfered with its free flow; the clumps had to be removed. This, in turn, significantly reduced the amount of blood left to transfuse. Before administering the blood, some physicians would stir it with a whisk or eggbeater to force the clumps to form, and then they would remove them. In the last half of the nineteenth century, physicians at Johns Hopkins would collect blood in Erlenmeyer flasks containing glass beads, which would cause the blood to clot, and thus make it easier to remove by filtering.[19] Another way around the problem was to try substituting milk or a saline solution as an alternative to blood.

As it became clear that animal blood was incompatible with human blood, the focus of physicians narrowed to transfusion solely between humans. The technique used in the nineteenth century was called the "direct method," which was a procedure used in Memphis as elsewhere in which the donor's artery was exposed surgically and connected to the recipient's exposed vein, either by suturing or by a cannula (a short length of tube). The advantage of this method was that it allowed a direct flow to the recipient, while avoiding clumping or any mixture of air. However, the procedure required skilled surgeons and numerous staff assistants. It also meant that the donor and recipient had to be in very close physical proximity to each other. Because of this arrangement, the outcome rested on the surgeon's judgment as to how much blood had been transfused, because there was no way to measure how much blood passed from the donor to the recipient.[20]

The history of blood banking in the twentieth century began with the intersection of three innovations. The first was the centuries-long desire by physicians to understand the nature of blood and its role in the body. Karl Landsteiner's discovery of blood types around 1900 gave an understanding of the composition of blood that made transfusion predictably safe.[21] Diggs sometimes liked to emphasize how well chosen his career as a hematologist was by pointing out that he was born in the same year as Landsteiner's discovery. The second innovation involved the availability of equipment, such as rubber tubing, flasks, rubber stoppers, and stopcocks (valves), which controlled the flow of blood in a more convenient and safe way. The third innovation was the realization that sodium citrate could be used as an anticoagulant, which eliminated the problem of clotting while the blood was in storage. Along with refrigeration, this ensured the preservation of blood for a week to ten days at a time.[22]

With these three innovations readily available, blood transfusion centers became possible. The first continuously operating blood bank in the United States was opened at the Mayo Clinic in 1935.[23] Subsequently, in 1937, a blood bank was established in the Cook County Hospital in Chicago, followed by others in Philadelphia and Los Angeles.[24] In this remarkable context, the first blood bank in the South was opened in Memphis at the John Gaston Hospital on Monday, April 25, 1938. At this time Memphis had the highest mortality rate among women in childbirth of any city in the country. The majority of women who developed bleeding during labor and delivery bled to death.[25] This fact, together with the shortage of blood in all areas of the hospital, made a blood bank a compelling need. It would store blood for immediate use, eliminate the confusion of contacting and typing potential donors, allow serum to be separated for use long after the shelf life of whole blood was past, reduce hospital expenses, and represent pioneering work in blood therapy.[26]

Diggs saw the need for and sought permission to create a blood bank in the John Gaston Hospital in Memphis. As a patient-oriented physician researcher, he was known to say that the goal of medicine should be to make "maximum use of our resources to make as many people as productive, as pain-free, and as happy as possible for as long as possible."[27] Diggs conceived of the idea after hearing about the blood bank at the Cook County Hospital a year earlier. He traveled to Chicago and learned about the operation of the unit, which relied on a system of donations and withdrawals; this process reminded the organizer Bernard Fantus of how a bank worked, and for this reason Fantus coined the term "blood bank." Since volunteers would continuously replenish the blood that was used, the only cost to the hospital would be supplies, which the hospital decided to assume. As long a relative or volunteer replaced the used blood, there was no charge to the patient. With this knowledge, Diggs returned to Memphis where, with the approval of the chief of surgery, Lucius McGehee, and the chief resident in surgery, Charles Olim, he began assembling the resources that were needed for starting a blood bank.[28]

The purchase of a special refrigerator represented a significant start-up expense. The Gaston Hospital was a city institution that operated with physicians, nurses, interns, and medical students from the University of Tennessee Medical Units. Since the city considered blood transfusions a laboratory expense, and the city's contract with the university designated such costs as state expenses, the university covered them. The start-up cost, equipment, and facilities were to come from both institutions. When Diggs realized that neither the city nor the state had the approximately two thousand dollars needed for the blood bank, he decided to make a public appeal.[29] At a meeting at the YMCA, Diggs made an extraordinary appeal to a group of Memphis businessmen, a plea that was heard by the local philanthropist Herbert Herff and members of the Temple Men's Club. Together they provided the money to procure the refrigerator and operating supplies.

Some in the Tennessee state capital considered this appeal to be an act of faculty disloyalty because Diggs went outside the state university system for financial support. Fortunately, the rebuke for his actions was mild. Diggs recounted: "Herbert Herff voluntarily and quite promptly obtained from a group of his Jewish friends in Memphis several thousand dollars which were used to purchase needed equipment, which included a new microscope, a large water-bath, ultra-violet lights for the processing room, and a four-door storage refrigerator with a recording thermometer and red signal lights that automatically flashed in the hall when there was electrical or motor failure."[30] The Memphis chapter of the Red Cross also provided funding for the position of a medical technician (someone who would train other personnel) for a period of six months. The new blood bank was located on the sixth floor of the hospital but was later relocated to the first floor to make access easier for donors.

The accepted practice concerning the supply of blood in Memphis and elsewhere before 1938 was to rely on family members and friends for blood to transfuse. However, in 1938 there were no black donors who volunteered to donate, despite public appeals to them and the large number of black patients in the John Gaston Hospital.[31] Elsewhere, professional donors were used, and hospitals paid for their donations on demand. This was true at other Memphis hospitals, but not at the Gaston Hospital, probably because of the difficulty of finding reliable professional donors and the lack of funds for paying them. The process of finding blood donors from family and friends that were compatible with a given patient's blood was time consuming, often requiring the testing of six or more donors before finding a suitable one. The effort could require as many as twelve hours. With this much time passing, it was not unusual for the patient to bleed to death before the process could be completed. It also assumed that the patient had family support in order to make donations a possibility.[32]

Relying on family and friends for potential donors mitigated concerns about the race of the donor or what might happen if blood was transfused across races. The patient would know the origin of the blood, and this knowledge minimized the issue of race. However, when blood banking started in 1938, the donor in effect was moved out of the picture. Now, when a patient and his or her family faced a decision about the use of blood from someone unknown to the patient, the situation reemphasized the role of race. Patients had to be informed before the transfusion took place as to where the blood came from; perhaps they were also given some of the donor's personal information. The patient was allowed to make the decision and sign a form either to accept or to reject the blood. Some patients did reject blood on the grounds that it was from the "wrong" race, but the patient could refuse it for any reason, including religious or political ones. As Diggs recalled, "Occasionally Baptists refused to receive blood from Methodists, Protestants from Catholics and in rare instances because of their religion, parents of children or patients preferred to risk death rather than to allow transfusion."[33]

Located in the Jim Crow South, the blood bank operated from the beginning under the assumption that the city would segregate black and white blood in its hospital. This was most likely a continuation and formalization of the practice that had prevailed when only direct transfusions were given. The ease and rapid accessibility of the new technology emphasized the separation of all blood units by race. Some medical personnel approved this decision, in part because of their own prejudices. But they also had concerns that the new bank would not work as well as expected. For example, there were some who felt that transfused cold blood would be toxic. Others were concerned that infectious diseases could be transmitted to the patient, and the perception was that the greater risk lay in black rather than in white blood: "Because of the high incidence of syphilis among blacks and the inadequate treatment which they receive, preliminary Kline precipitation test are performed by their laboratory interns on all negroes before they are selected as donors. After the blood for transfusion is collected in the bank, a check Kahn test is run in the serologic laboratory. White donors are questioned about primary and secondary lesions, blood tests and previous treatment, but preliminary tests for syphilis are not made before the bloods are taken. It has been found by experience that few bloods from white donors are discarded because of positive serology."[34] The Kahn test was a widely recognized and inexpensive blood test for syphilis.[35]

In 1937, the John Gaston Hospital was treating three thousand to four thousand cases of syphilis, and the psychiatric clinic was full of patients suffering from neurosyphilis: "The treatment of syphilis consisted of 30 weekly injections of an arsenical and 40 of a bismuth preparation, given in alternating courses over a period of one and a half years. To achieve noninfectiousness required a minimum of 20 injections of each." [36] Not surprisingly, when a study was done, it was found that less than 15 percent of patients receiving treatment completed their course of injections. It was estimated that about 30 percent of the black population had some form of the disease, which affected a significant but smaller percentage of the white population. Treatment of the disease was hampered by the lack of an effective medicine (penicillin would not be used widely until about 1943, the year that the disease peaked in Memphis) and the social silence that shrouded references to the disease. The Kahn test would have detected the presence of the disease in potential donors and thus kept the rate of syphilis transmissions at an acceptably low level.

Although the hospital segregated blood and hospital staff informed patients about the blood that was available for transfusion, some hospital personnel, Diggs among them, believed that there was no biological difference or medical justification for this separation by race. They believed that, as long as blood types were compatible, transfusion could proceed without any consideration of race. However, at this time in American medicine, some medical personnel believed that there existed a physical and detectable difference between black and white bloods. Historian Keith Wailoo has shown that from the 1920s to the 1940s many believed that blood analysis offered insights into salient questions of racial identity and hereditary character, beginning with the discovery of sickle cell anemia and of Emmel's technique to produce sickled cells (which demonstrated latency to sickling that was thought to be characteristic of black blood only). People also believed that sickle cell was unique to blacks and that the few cases found among whites were the result of earlier cross-racial relationships. As Wailoo observed, "For many physicians in the early twentieth century, *Negro blood* was a term with clear technological origins and with biological, social, and public health meanings. These physicians based their view on what was at that time hematological evidence and scientific understanding of the genetics of the disorder."[37] The Red Cross also segregated its blood at this time and drew heavy criticism from those disagreeing with its policy, such as the American Association of Physical Anthropologists in 1942 and afterward.[38]

In 1941, in a Sunday edition of the Memphis *Commercial Appeal*, an article of over two full pages on the Gaston Hospital's blood bank emphasized the separation of blood by race and its rigid enforcement. The reporter explained the reason for separation: "Scientifically, according to the doctors, the blood of one race will serve quite satisfactorily for transfusion to a person of a different race. But there are other considerations. One of them is that since Negro patients are in the majority at John Gaston, it is only just that Negro donors should furnish their proper share of blood; and that white patients, in the minority, should receive their blood from white donors. In short, that each race should provide its own needs. In this way any question of racial discrimination has been avoided."[39] Despite the acknowledgment by the author that there may be no scientific reason for separation, he cites "other considerations" for maintaining the separation of blood without elaborating on what they might be.

Despite the findings of medicine and science, southern custom still dictated the separation of black and white blood. The reporter used a financial metaphor to suggest that blood, like money, must be paid and used in a strictly regulated way, with each donor and each recipient paying his or her own way. In reality, however, the rigid separation of blood was carried out only in principle. In practice, if the need arose, a patient was offered blood from the other race, with the clear understanding that the patient could refuse the blood if he or she chose to do so and was willing to sign a waiver to that effect. Diggs wrote, "From a scientific point of view there is no justification for drawing a color line in the blood bank, but the presence of sentiment, and prejudice in the matter on the part of the patients cannot be denied. When in emergencies blood of one race is used for another, the patient or some responsible member of his family gives permission in writing."[40]

In other words, the public policy expressed in the newspaper was not exactly the same as that practiced in the clinic. As long as the donor and the recipient were typed and matched properly, the transfusion would be successful. Diggs knew this and, despite his resistance to the idea of segregating bloods, he implemented the policy to segregate by race.[41] Blood donations were stored in bottles with labels indicating the name, blood type, and race of the donor, and a two-column file card organizer with "white" at the top of one column and "black" at the top of the other recorded what units were available by type and who had donated. However, strict enforcement of the separation of blood was not maintained within the storage refrigerator. Photographs of the refrigerator and its contents show several bottles on a shelf of the refrigerator; a close inspection of the labels reveals that at least one bottle with "black" circled on the label stands next to a bottle with the word "white" circled on its label. That this was a deliberate and normal practice in contrast to stated hospital policy seems clear.[42]

At first, other hospitals in Memphis did not react to the opening of the blood bank. Gaston was a public hospital while all the others were private. The patient population of Gaston consisted predominantly of black citizens from the Mid-South while the private hospitals were exclusively white. Since Gaston was the first of its kind in Memphis and the South, and the blood bank's benefits gradually became obvious, it took only a few years before Baptist and St. Joseph's hospitals followed with their own blood banks.[43] It was characteristic of blood banks in these early years that only hospitals opened them, and this would remain true even as the Second World War exerted a powerful influence on the national blood supply.[44] Given the immediate need that hospitals had for blood products, their medical expertise, and their control of operating costs, hospitals were in an advantageous situation. Because hospital blood banks were considered an internal resource, they had few, if any, incentives to collaborate with each other. In the case of the John Gaston Hospital, it soon became apparent that the blood bank would have an even greater significance than initially thought. Since it was a public hospital with patients from Tennessee, Mississippi, and Arkansas, and because it played an obvious role in community disasters, such as tornados, epidemics, and storms, the need to store blood became a regional rather than simply citywide necessity. As the need for blood transfusions increased, Diggs began enlarging the blood bank's operation.[45]

Apart from the issue of race, effectively staffing and equipping the facility was still a practical consideration. No companies existed to produce the bottles, stoppers, tubing, and other supplies, and no one taught the process of blood banking. Diggs had to rely on his own expertise and best judgment. From 1939 to 1941 he began publishing a series of articles on blood banks, in which he shared not only what types of physical layout and administrative structure worked well, but where the mistakes were, how they were resolved, and what could be learned from them.[46]

When the Gaston blood bank opened, Diggs found that the best time for drawing blood was on weekdays, from 6:00 to 10:00 p.m., after people had left work. However, in practice, anyone could make a blood donation at any time of the day. The blood bank staff selected only family members and friends of patients as donors and did not use professional donors. Although the unit had Diggs as a clinical pathologist and a nurse supervisor as full-time personnel, the staff also included interns, medical students, nursing students, and technology students. The advantage of students was that they were plentiful and capable of performing the required tasks, which compensated for their main disadvantage, that they rotated through the unit as part of their educational duties and were always relatively inexperienced.[47]

One of the first lessons that Diggs learned was that the prolonged shelf life of blood units allowed more time for contamination of the blood by bacteria. Earlier, blood was taken from the donor by allowing it to drain from the donor's arm through an open-ended tube into an open, uncovered container with sodium citrate as an anticoagulant. The practice was based on the idea that a blood donation would be transfused almost immediately into the recipient, and thus contamination by elements in the air was minimal. The first ten or so blood units drawn after the new blood bank had opened were tested, found to be contaminated after a few days, and discarded as a result. For this reason, Diggs switched to a closed, sterilized system that included bottles with two-hole rubber stoppers that would minimize exposure to the air.[48]

The realization that cooler temperatures preserved blood was an important step on the road to blood banking. Diggs found that blood could typically be stored at one to six degrees Celsius. Together with sodium citrate as an anticoagulant, he could keep blood safely and reliably for a week to ten days. At first he believed that, before the blood could be transfused, it would have to be warmed, or the cold blood would result in a reaction by the patient. However, with experience, it became clear that it was unnecessary to warm the blood, because there were no reactions by patients, and, it turned out, the process of warming the blood could lead to overheating and a destruction of red cells that would induce a reaction in the patient. The worst that happened, Diggs found, in the transfusion of cold blood was a cooling sensation in the recipient's arm, but the recipient's core body temperature remained unaltered.[49]

Diggs also explored issues related to needle size and placement. His concern was first to determine the size of the needle that would be most efficient for drawing blood from the donor's arm. For some time, the 13-gauge needle was considered best because of its larger diameter. However, 14- and 15-gauge needles were smaller and worked well in men and women, without extending the donation time (and the insertion of these smaller needles proved less painful for the patients). The even smaller 16-gauge needle took longer to draw the blood, and he thus excluded it from recommendation. Another concern for Diggs was the placement of the needle in the arm, which was usually in the direction of venous blood flow, toward the shoulder. Diggs and his staff considered whether it would accelerate the process if the needle were inserted in the arm against venous flow, toward the hand instead, to see if this placement shortened the withdrawal time by meeting the flow of blood "head on." It did not, because the pressure in the vein was the same, regardless of needle direction. Still another consideration was whether negative pressure by mouth or by machine in the flask could be used to draw the blood from the body more quickly. But the added cost in terms of technology and skill, not to mention the possibility of collapsed veins in the patient, made this idea unacceptable.[50]

For one year after the opening of the Memphis blood bank, Erlenmeyer flasks were used to collect blood, but the cost of the flasks and the awkwardness of the triangular shape of the bottle for storage led Diggs to consider another solution. Always looking for a way to cut costs by simplifying matters, he thought of the idea of using milk bottles instead. The refrigerator was filling up with donated blood, and he could see that the triangular flasks were inefficient for the space in the compartment. In comparison, the parallel sides of the milk bottles could fit tightly together and increase the number of units that could be stored. In addition to being cheaper, the bottles had large mouths that fit the rubber stoppers used in the hospital, and they could be easily sterilized for reuse. Diggs put the milk bottles into use in 1939, and they were used for more than three years afterwards.[51]

Diggs exercised creativity in using the clinical supplies that were available to the hospital for the new blood bank, but he possessed a notable inventive streak as well. During the donation process, while the intern was drawing the blood from the donor, a second person continuously shook the bottle receiving the blood. Sodium citrate prevented the blood from coagulating, and the shaking mixed the citrate uniformly with the blood; because blood coagulates when it stops moving, the shaking provided additional anticoagulation. However, shaking is a mechanical process that can just as easily be accomplished by a machine as by a person. Jeanette Spann, who had been hired in 1938, was the first full-time medical technologist. She contributed to the idea of a mechanical shaker that would inhibit the tendency of blood to clump after being drawn. Colin F. Vorder Bruegge, at the time a medical student working in the blood bank, "used a universal joint from a Model T Ford and a discarded disc player"[52] to design the first shaker. Later Dr. Vorder Bruegge became brigadier general in the U.S. Army and director of the Armed Forces Institute of Pathology. Subsequently, Diggs sought help in building the device. He turned for help to J. M. Smith and his students at the newly opened William R. Moore School of Technology in Memphis. Together they designed a machine, using an electric motor from a Victrola phonograph attached to an eccentric disk that would gently shake the bottles during the course of the donation.[53] Two years later, Diggs implemented an improved design. This new device not only made the task of shaking the bottle easier, but it also meant that the task of drawing blood from a donor henceforth could be managed by a single person.[54]

The opportunities for pioneering work in the blood bank were not lost on the technologists working in it. A part-time technologist, Alice Jean Keith, developed a simple cross-matching technique, which consisted of "dipping a wooden applicator stick into the blood clot of a donor and transferring a few red cells to a glass slide containing a drop of serum from the recipient."[55] The slide could then be examined microscopically for compatibility. This procedure proved to be safe "before the Rh and other less common blood factors were known and before testing by the Coombs procedure came into use."[56] Spann also took advantage of circumstances to find new ways to store sterile needles, and she contributed to the design of blood collection tables with sliding and sloping arm boards, wire springs to prevent kinking in tubes, and metal filters and special needle adapters with wide lumens.

In these early years, only hospitals opened blood banks for internal use. There existed no regulatory authorities to oversee the operation of the blood bank in Memphis or elsewhere. The protocols for operation were based on the experience and ethics of the physicians in charge. There were no regional or national organizations that took up this cause until the war in Europe appeared to be unavoidable, at which time the American Red

Cross initiated a national crusade. The war and its prospect of wounded and dying soldiers more than justified a national campaign to raise awareness of the importance of a national blood supply.[57] Although the Gaston blood bank participated in American Red Cross drives and the larger involvement in the war, its primary focus continued as a local and regional resource. Eventually the other Memphis hospitals began operation of their own blood banks, and it is clear that money was available to support the increased demand for storage and the hiring of personnel. By this time, reciprocal agreements were also in place to assure that the Gaston blood bank had adequate supplies.[58]

The growth of the blood bank in number of transfusions given is astonishing. In June of 1937 a report to Memphis mayor Watkins Overton's office for that month indicated that 87 blood transfusions had taken place, about 1,000 for the year, all at the John Gaston Hospital.[59] By 1941 the number of transfusions jumped to 200 per month, about 2,400 per year.[60] By 1950 the Gaston Hospital and the four major hospitals in the city were giving 18,000–20,000 transfusions annually.[61] This exponential increase was a clear sign that blood banking had become an indisputable asset to healthcare in the area; undoubtedly this change was further magnified by the United States' experience during World War II.

By 1942, Diggs's reputation as an expert on blood transfusion and banking was being recognized in the local press. He recognized the importance of blood banks for normal and wartime conditions, noting that blood reserves were inadequate even for peacetime disasters and criticizing the hospital community for not meeting this challenge. At a meeting of the Memphis Pubic Affairs Forum on February 2, he spoke on the subject of the city's disaster preparedness. He began his remarks by asking, "What is being done about blood plasma as a defense measure in Memphis?" After a pause, he responded, "I know the answer. Nothing is being done."[62] There are plenty of donors, he told the audience, but the need was for expanded facilities and some specialized equipment, such as refrigerators. The need was not hypothetical, because there had been an explosion in nearby Millington a few days before. One month later, about one hundred victims needed transfusions after tornados struck in Kentucky, Tennessee, and Mississippi. "We had enough blood in storage to take care of at least 100 victims. But if there had been several hundred victims, we would have lacked facilities for taking blood from Memphis hospitals to some other point where it would be needed immediately."[63] A worse tornado that occurred one year earlier would have overwhelmed the blood bank. If an appeal to the community worked once before, as it did in getting the refrigerator needed for equipping the Gaston blood bank, then perhaps it would work this time, too. And it did. Within a few weeks, the "astounded" audience galvanized itself. As it was reported in the *Memphis Press-Scimitar,* "Two meetings of civic leaders, superintendents of hospitals, physicians and Red Cross workers have already been held—and in a month or six weeks the facilities that Dr. Diggs and others have hoped for will be fully provided."[64] The hospitals were beginning to work together, and the American Red Cross announced that it would supply plasma should an enemy attack the city. "More than 55,000 civilians have donated blood since the Pearl Harbor attack—and in about a month from now, when facilities are ready in Memphis, many more Memphis donors will be added to this number."[65]

Four years after the Gaston Hospital blood bank opened, Baptist, St. Joseph's, and other hospitals opened or expanded their own units for local use.[66] World War II added impetus to the need for banks for whole blood and for serum, but the focus continued to be local and regional. By 1942, the Gaston Hospital bank was already beginning to struggle to keep up with the growth and change elsewhere. "We have asked for those facilities . . . but at the present time the hospital budget is not prepared to meet the cost and the $4000 or $5000 needed would have to be provided by special action of the City Commission."[67] Once again the limited budgets of the city and the state made keeping up with technological changes very difficult. Diggs stated in a newspaper article, "John Gaston hardly is able to maintain enough blood and plasma for normal needs, and never has any plasma ahead."[68]

In a manner characteristic of his intellectual style, Diggs set out to create a knowledge base for blood banking and blood transfusion in general, as he had for sickle cell anemia. With his encouragement, the Zonta Club in Memphis began identifying and assembling reprints of every medical article pertaining to blood banking, including those by foreign doctors. It did not take long before there were over five hundred articles filed in the John Gaston blood bank office that were available free to anyone who wanted to learn more about the subject. At this time there was little known among the general population about this process, and this repository was to serve as a resource for anyone with an interest in learning more about it.[69] This collection also served Diggs's desire to become knowledgeable about all aspects of blood banking and transfusion. On May 4, 1942, he presented a detailed history of blood transfusion to a nonmedical after-dinner audience at the faculty banquet at the University of Mississippi in Oxford.

The segregation of black and white bloods continued to be a national issue, and it was hotly debated in the medical as well as the popular media.[70] The objection to segregating was that there simply was no medical reason for supporting the practice; as long as the blood units were properly matched, transfusion was predictably safe. In Memphis, without the glare of national prominence that accompanied the decisions and actions of the military, and despite the Red Cross's policy of segregation, the physicians, nurses, and technicians at the Gaston Hospital blood bank continued dealing with race until the problem was either resolved or became a non-issue. Diggs wrote, "A few years later, the 'Jim Crow Law' in the blood bank was ignored by mutual consent of all intelligent persons."[71] When precisely this separation of white and black blood came to an end is unclear, but Diggs and others accelerated its demise by simply dodging the issue until it faded away. Once he established the blood bank and reduced the process of drawing and transfusing blood to a routine that could be handled easily by technicians, it no longer required his supervision. His interest in sickle cell anemia continued, and the war years offered new opportunities that took him away from Memphis. As a result of Diggs's clear-sighted and concerted efforts, the blood bank continued to grow as a valuable resource for restoring the health of patients.

The task of implementing a blood bank in the Memphis general hospital was both easy and difficult. Diggs saw the medical and staffing feasibility of the bank, managed the cultural beliefs of the city, tried new ideas, and shared what he learned through his publications. It was not long before the concept of blood banking was widely accepted, and within ten years all city hospitals had one. After World War II, there was enough interest among the hospitals to form a community organization for sharing blood units that competed with the American Red Cross.[72]

Diggs's stature in the community and his reputation as a physician grew because of his sickle cell research and his interest in medical technology, especially his commitment to blood banking. From 1939 to 1943 he produced approximately thirteen publications on the techniques and problems associated with the subject. In one noteworthy article, he argued the practicality of training medical technologists for blood banks as well as laboratories as part of the medical school curriculum. In the years immediately following World War II, the economic condition of the nation had improved considerably, and medical schools were beginning to position themselves for the brighter period ahead. With his impressive reputation, Diggs received a number of offers to go to other schools. Although he was not predisposed to consider moving, he considered the offers, if only because he felt that he was not receiving the salary and recognition that were commensurate with his status in the profession, and because he realized that he needed to provide for his growing family.

$5 + 4 + 6 + 0 = 15$
$5 \times 4 \times 6 \times 0 = 0$
Let 0 = lack of spirituality

Chapter 4
World War II and the Cleveland Clinic

For the University of Tennessee Medical Units, World War II brought increased patient loads. The number of doctors declined as younger doctors went into the military while, at the same time, teaching loads increased. Diggs relinquished some control of the Gaston Hospital Blood Bank in the belief that the operation of the bank was sufficiently understood that it did not require a physician to coordinate; a nurse or a technician could manage it. His aim was not to distance himself from the blood bank as much as to make its operation a team effort with himself as the boss. The person assisting him was Jeanette Spann, whom Diggs hired in 1938 just after the blood bank opened.[1]

The war changed the atmosphere on campus, and the focus on military needs moved the campus in a new direction. Diggs had an interest in malaria as a blood disease, and the research effort was given over to supporting the needs of wartime diseases, including those likely to be found in the Pacific. Uniformed students permeated the student population, changing the look and tone of the campus. The uniforms represented mainly the

Army and the Navy. The quacking of ducks was what many people remembered from this time on campus.[2] As Diggs recalled, "At that time various drugs were being tried on ducks with avian malaria strains. We were also treating patients with CNS syphilis on mosquito inoculation with various strains of human and monkey malaria."[3] Monkeys were also used as part of the malaria research.

Pearl Harbor had galvanized the nation, and the focus of research and education at the Medical Units was directed wherever possible to support military needs. Despite its local focus, the Gaston blood bank worked together with the Red Cross to answer the call for blood products, especially for plasma. Plasma had a much longer shelf life than whole blood, and when freeze-dried it lasted indefinitely and needed only distilled water to reconstitute it. There was no need for typing or matching of donors and recipients; any recipient could receive plasma from any donor, which is what made it so valuable in peacetime or war. The technique for the mass processing and shipping of dried plasma was the innovation of Charles Drew, a noted black physician at a time when blood was segregated in blood banks.[4]

One of Diggs's first assignments of the war years was his selection in 1943 as a Markle Foundation[5] Fellow in Tropical Medicine through the Association of American Medical Colleges to Guatemala and El Salvador, where his task was to study tropical diseases in preparation for teaching medical personnel.[6] The medical experience was eye-opening. He was trained to understand malaria as it occurred in Central America. It had been epidemic at times but had been brought under control by the elimination of standing water, which bred the mosquitoes that carried the parasite. What he found in Quiriguá, the first Guatemalan city he visited, was an excellent laboratory that he could use as a base for his investigations. The most obvious feature of the location was that malaria was so pervasive that the medical staff were inclined to diagnose every case that came into the hospital as malaria until proven otherwise: "Malaria in the Montagua Valley is so common and so deadly that they treat all patients for it regardless of the laboratory, and after seeing patients die of blackwater fever and cerebral malaria, I am convinced that their way is best for the area."[7] However, the inclination to call everything malaria meant that it "dulls their suspicion for other diseases."[8] Diggs felt that some of the "anemias, splenomegalies [enlarged spleens], jaundices, heart murmurs, and pains" could have other explanations, but there was little interest in differential diagnoses. Patient histories were not taken, so records were not a source of much information for understanding malaria. He found that he was also hampered by his lack of Spanish skills as well as the different medical culture. All in all, he compared the organization to an industrial hospital: "Their aim was to look after the immediate acute sickness, to get the patient back to work as soon as possible and not to bother too much about details or exact diagnoses."[9]

The treatments for malaria were also of interest. Diggs found that calomel, a mercury compound, was used along with magnesium sulfate, atebrin, and plasmoquin compound, "followed by pink pills which contain a little quinine, arsenic, iron, and nux vomica."[10] "Blackwaters[11] are treated by keeping in hot blankets to encourage sweating and copious fluids (water, barley water, citrus fruit juices, and Sternberg's solution). Drugs given are Vit. C, caffeine, sedatives if necessary and horse serum. I could not see the rationale for the horse serum, but they seemed content to follow routine and seemed to get irritated when I questioned any procedures. No food was given until the patient began to void freely. I followed hematocrits on some of the patients and found that they developed a severe anemia very rapidly with very little regenerative response on the part of the bone marrow."[12] Diggs learned about the striking array of drugs that were used to treat malaria and in what combinations. He saw little or no evidence of sickle cell anemia during his trip.

Overall the trip was not unpleasant, and it was a learning experience for Diggs and the other fellows: "The visits to hospitals, medical schools, clinics, etc., were mainly impressive in showing us how far they have to go and how backward is public health in C.A. [Central America]."[13] Characteristically, Diggs explored "behind the ditches, the people, their housing, manner of living and nutrition, in order to visualize the magnitude of the problem, the lack of support to be expected from the native population and the difficulties."[14] In his report to the American Association of Medical Colleges, he added, "The opportunity for us to widen our horizon, to see that public health is not a matter of a city or county but of countries working together was appreciated."[15] And it was well within this belief that he saw medicine as a social need that could perhaps be best served by organizations such as governments getting involved, a feeling that was also reinforced by his experience treating sickle cell patients in Memphis.

Diggs saw a social system in Guatemala in which the lack of access to healthcare or the means to afford it had a detrimental affect on the people and their country. Diggs believed that all organizations, social or political, ought to be based on the personal responsibility of the individuals that form the groups, whether social, professional, or political, and that members of the groups should be individually responsible for their organizations' actions. Individuals contribute to and form organizations for the benefit of individuals, which are constitutive of any group. In part this belief was formed as a young man growing up in Virginia. Diggs read works by the country's founding fathers, including George Mason, who wrote the first drafts of the Virginia Declaration of Rights and the Virginia Constitution, both of 1776, and Thomas Paine, whose deistic conviction as well as political rhetoric in *Common Sense* influenced Diggs's thinking on human and civil rights.[16]

Diggs's view of personal responsibility as the basis for any group or organization was also reflected in his acceptance of Unitarianism and his philosophy of science. Although born and raised in a strict Methodist family, after high school and leaving home he began to move away from his family's religion. After moving to Memphis, Diggs and his wife, Beatrice, joined the Unitarian Universalist Church, with its rejection of the traditional Christian concept of a Trinity, the godhood of Jesus, or any "fixed dogma" or "any authority as the ultimate truth."[17] Diggs did believe in a higher power, and his conception of religion also correlated with his view of science. His religion explicitly believed that "The universe is meaningful" and that "the laws of nature (laws of God) are established, can be depended upon and always work the same way."[18] What tied science and religion together for Diggs was his belief that "Man is given intelligence and is expected to use his head."[19] Both the intellect and the soul must grow: "To the extent that he can discover the laws of nature and adopt his living to these laws the better he adjusts and gets along. This applies not only to disease, but to social, economic and political problems."[20] His beliefs are also a reflection of his upbringing and early readings.[21]

Diggs held to these beliefs throughout his career, although did not write much about them. In 1943, however, a Tennessee State College professor asked Diggs in a letter about his views on religion and science. In response, Diggs declared that "there is no conflict between science and Christianity."[22] He explained it this way: "The consideration of the universe through the telescope reveals a magnitude that awes us and the revelations of the microscope reveal a smallness that is likewise big. In the advances of chemistry are revealed molecular structures comparable to the stars. Anyone who is a scientist has to admit the presence of a controlling power over things and the existence of a spiritual universe that is greater than his."[23] The world has meaning, Diggs seems to be saying, because the universe was created with a complexity and organization that could be discerned by anyone willing to make the effort—an organization and complexity that could only have been created by a higher being.

But, in Diggs's religion, individuals can understand the world they live in without the need for a religious organization to make sense of it for them. Indeed, religious organizations that insist on adherence to a system of beliefs only perpetuate misunderstanding and discourage inquiry: "The acceptance of Christ as a man and as an inspiration is entirely compatible with science but the oriental interpretations of heaven and hell and immortality and essential sin are opinions of man recorded years ago and misinterpreted through the centuries. To insist upon them as divine truths is to weaken the church and to drive away from it intelligent people and to keep the others from thinking."[24] The individual is his or her own best guide to understanding the world he or she lived in while still living in a community of people, with each possessing the freedom to accept or reject the ideas discussed within that community. Diggs summarized the core of his belief in this way: "I personally believe that a search after truth and the application of truth to living is the best form of religion."[25]

If the war stirred an interest in research at the UT Medical Units, it also afforded Diggs as head of the Clinical Pathology Department the opportunity to hire a secretary to help attend to his correspondence, writing, and record keeping. In 1942 he hired Ann Bell, a young woman who had been born and raised in Memphis and completed her bachelor's degree at Randolph-Macon Women's College in Lynchburg, Virginia. After graduation she returned to Memphis. She was attracted to science and found a secretarial position at the Medical Units. Apart from nursing, the medical professions offered few opportunities to women. Laboratory workers were needed to do routine tests, and the field of medical technology had grown since the beginning of the century. The first woman to graduate with a medical degree from the Medical Units was in 1913, and others followed, but their numbers were always small and the path to graduation was much more difficult than for their male counterparts.

On the other hand, medical technology was one of the few entrées into the healthcare field that was advertised as appropriate for women, even if that recommendation was based on the stereotype of women as better at accuracy and attention to detail. However, what drove the profession's growth was the war, which attracted so many technicians into the military that there was a demand to replace them in hospitals like Gaston. Although Diggs advocated the creation of a medical technology program, the chief executive of the Medical Units, O. W. Hyman, refused to implement the proposal due to limited means. Consequently, many technologists were trained as apprentices. Diggs relied on the laboratory and was always on the lookout for good, dependable laboratory workers.[26] Although Bell began work as a secretary, it soon became clear that she wanted to do more and that her interest was in the laboratory, so Diggs trained her in laboratory techniques from 1942 to 1947. Very quickly he came to depend on her skill and dedication. Local musician Roosevelt Jamison also learned laboratory technique as an apprentice to Diggs. Jazz historian Peter Guralnick gives this account: "Though the University of Tennessee was strictly segregated at the time, Diggs began taking Roosevelt to lectures as his slide projectionist and then quizzing him on the content of the lectures in private. In this way Roosevelt came to be certified as a medical technologist, . . ." [27] How many Diggs cultivated in this way is not known.

Within a few months of his visit to Central America, Diggs and his family were in Rochester, New York, where he took a temporary position to replace his former teacher at the University of Rochester, William McCann, who was on military leave to the Navy. The war had increased research and educational demands across the country and, like many, Diggs was interested to see what the employment opportunities would be like elsewhere in light of the situation he found in Memphis and despite his promotion to associate professor in 1938. Along with the Markle Foundation Fellowship, Diggs spent time "as a physician for one summer with DuPont at the time this company was manufacturing explosive materials."[28]

The return to the University of Rochester must have felt like a homecoming for Diggs and his wife. Diggs had met and trained his future wife there, and it was Beatrice's hometown. As Diggs related, "We have a convenient and comfortable apartment or rather apartments, for we are in part living with Mother Moshier and have a two room apartment in addition. After living at Whitehaven I feel like a caged animal and feel sorry for the kids."[29]

But much had changed. His work focused on the hematological changes in cats following the surgical removal of adrenal glands. He was also able to do "comparative studies of stained blood smears and of moist preparations stained by supravital dyes."[30] He wrote to Ann Bell in Memphis that his office had only standard equipment and "a place to hang my hat,"[31] and it was across the hall from the student labs. He conducted weekday morning rounds for the students, and case studies three times per week. The case studies were diagnostic exercises "with a lot of x-ray, lab, E.K.G. all done, so it is very interesting as well as challenging." The students asked questions, which included one or two that "you do not know but should."[32] Ann Bell was his lifeline, helping him to maintain communications with colleagues in Memphis and sending him items as needed.

The situation at the University of Rochester contrasted with the circumstances in Memphis. Diggs's schedule was not so full that he could not spend time in the library perusing the medical literature. It also allowed him time to prepare his promised lectures to the students and faculty on sickle cell anemia, malaria, and the treatment of anemias, for which Ann sent the slides as he needed them. Although he saw no sickle cell patients during this period, he did receive slides from the Army showing the presence of sickle cell in a white patient. The circumstances of sickle cell appearing in this patient are not known, but the announcement of a nonblack occurrence of the disease added to what he already knew, namely that the disease was not limited to African Americans. Ann also sent him patent forms for a blood transfusion device, probably an updated version of the bottle shaker used in the Memphis blood bank. She had O. W. Hyman fill in part of the form before forwarding it to Diggs. He filed the papers with the U.S. Patent Office to register a collection, storage, and transfusion bottle with the stopper assembly attached to the mouth of a milk bottle. The patent was granted on February 10, 1948.[33] He was also working up an article on the blood picture in malaria. By the beginning of September he was reaching the end of his stay in Rochester. On September 8, Beatrice and the children returned by train to Memphis while Diggs stayed behind to complete his remaining courses. Then he went on to Hampton, Virginia, to visit his mother before returning to Memphis.

He noted that the fall was just beginning when he left Rochester and the weather was comfortable in Memphis, where he had a few months to orient himself for what he thought would be a permanent move to Ohio in January 1945, where he had accepted an offer to join the faculty of the Cleveland Clinic. The move was an opportunity for Diggs to work at a prestigious medical center, probably including a significant salary increase, but his plans may also have been tactical as well as practical. He hedged his bets by maintaining ties with his Memphis friends and colleagues. He had been struggling with his low salary and was looking for some way to raise it. It seemed clear that he could not do so by staying at the University of Tennessee, so he chose the time-honored option of moving to another institution. The family knew that Diggs was making the move for financial reasons, but he told at least some of his colleagues in Memphis that he was leaving because clinical pathology was not receiving enough recognition at the university and there were better opportunities to practice in the field at the Cleveland Clinic.[34] Probably both reasons were part of this thinking.

If fall had only just arrived in Rochester, by the time Diggs reached Cleveland a full-fledged winter had arrived to greet him. The snow and ice complicated his search for an apartment. As he related, "Having arrived in a blizzard, waded around up to knees in snow drifts looking for a room without success and obliterated a few capillaries in my ears from the cold, have decided to stay in a hotel until the sun shines again and the sidewalks show up."[35] For a man raised in the South who probably envisioned spending his career there, the arrival in Cleveland was no doubt a challenge, if not a demanding one.

The situation at the Cleveland Clinic looked promising. Dr. Russell Haden was a consummate researcher there and the longtime chair of the Division of Medicine. He had been division head, supervised the clinical laboratories, and carried a heavy clinical load. In 1944 he gave up supervising the clinical laboratories and created the Department of Clinical Pathology, to which he appointed Diggs as head. Diggs became head of the department without being formally designated as its chair.[36]

Diggs was excited at the opportunity. His new office would be located on the same floor where "major interesting hematology is done by Dr. Haden's research staff of three full-time technicians, so [I] will be in the middle of the activity [I] am most interested in."[37] He saw the opportunities to learn more about megakaryocytes[38] in a better setting, and he found the staff friendly. He could focus on his research and teaching in a way that most satisfied him. The highlight of his stay at the Cleveland Clinic was the opportunity to review the "coverslip preparations of bone marrows with excellent accompanying and follow-up records."[39] By being given access to Dr. Haden's work, Diggs was able to draw conclusions that led to publications related to "Idiopathic Thrombocytopenic Purpura, Plasma Cell Myeloma, Hodgkin's Disease, cytology of cells in bronchial washings, tests employed in hemorrhagic diseases and methods employed in sedimentation tests."[40] His unpublished papers from this period were on topics such as metastatic cells in bone marrow, leukocyte counts, and differentials in association with jaundice. According to Diggs, "Many of the men here are experts in their field and it is stimulating to be associated with them. At the clinical conferences they do not hesitate to jump on each other critically before the group for the sake of the patient. At the X ray conference this afternoon, they showed plates and made the fellows in turn get up in front of his associates and stick his neck out as to what he saw in skull or lung or kidney plate; teaching in the raw and most revealing for those not so well trained."[41]

Diggs found the environment at the Cleveland Clinic challenging in a way that he did not experience in Memphis. He was also aware of the state the clinical laboratories were in and how much work he would have to do to improve them. Some of the Cleveland doctors had special interests, such as one with an interest in crystals in urine or the gastrointestinal clinic's preference for Ewald tubes, which Diggs considered outdated. All in all he was looking for places that needed improvement and procedures that could be simplified. He was also looking forward to time that could be spent in the library and in study. The malaria paper that he had hoped to complete in the fall was still "plugging along."[42] As in Rochester, Diggs continued to rely on Ann Bell for charts, forms, and mimeographs that would be helpful in his new position.

Diggs had the opportunity to establish a second blood bank at the Cleveland Clinic. It was probably his reputation as someone who had successfully started one in Memphis that led the Cleveland Clinic's administration to commission Diggs to build one on its premises. He modeled it on the one he designed in Memphis. The request was made several months earlier, while he was still at the University of Rochester. He requested Ann Bell to send reprints of the floor plans for the Gaston bank to the Cleveland Clinic's architects in St. Paul.

Diggs was busy, with new things happening every day. He learned about new procedures not done in Memphis as well as procedures done in

Memphis that were not done or performed inadequately in Cleveland: "Such is the advantage and the stimulus of moving."[43] In February he was still awaiting the completion of renovations to his office and for a secretary to assist him, but the work was a pleasant distraction from the snow and the six inches of ice on the sidewalks. By March 23 the family had arrived in Cleveland: "it is more like spring, but it is still snowing occasionally and no flowers are yet in bloom."[44]

By June, Diggs had a secretary, who reported to Ann that he seemed to be doing very well since "he seems to sing a lot!"[45] Singing to himself was Diggs's habit when he was happy. Another reason might have been his pleasure at having the help he needed for his many projects. The summer was busier than usual, in part because the clinic staff was distracted by vacations. By September the busy summer work subsided, and he reported to Ann that, even though his own work continued to be interesting, the family still did not like Cleveland, so he renewed his request for news from the Gaston Hospital and, as always, sent his greetings to the staff there.

In January 1947, winter once again cast a shadow over the Diggs family's situation in Cleveland. After six months, technicians were still in short supply: "We still have trouble getting trained technicians and our staff of 38 are getting married or moving at about the rate of 1–2 per month."[46] Moreover, he was losing the capable service by the new secretary, who announced that she was "going to the Pacific as a medical missionary (!)"[47] In a few months she would take her vows in her church and move to a leper colony in the South Pacific. He would be without an assistant again and leery of hiring a new one because of the amount of time and energy that it would take to train a new person and the worry that, once trained, the new person might leave soon anyway. In March he wrote to Ann: "I still do not have a secretary-technician, and have not taken chance on applicants so far. How about moving to Cleveland and being in my office again."[48]

He preferred a semirural setting, and with that in mind found a house in Bedford, Ohio, some twenty miles from the clinic. It included a few acres of land. His daughter Alice remembered it well: "We did have a lake on one side of the front yard. On the other side there was just a narrow strip of a metropolitan park and there was a stream, a tumbling creek, called Tinker's Creek, was on the other side."[49] The location seemed perfect for the family and for growing a garden. There were also hills and a nearby neighborhood. Diggs built a cart for his daughter that led to cart races down the neighborhood streets. In the summer they played baseball, and in the winter they learned to ski and skated. They also took walks into the park adjacent to their property where, on one occasion while walking through the woods, they came across an illegal alcohol still.

Generally, however, the situation was not working out as well as Diggs had hoped for his family: "The kids are enjoying the ice & snow, but 'B' hates it up here and seems to like it less as time goes on. I do not like such a large city but find my work stimulating and associations at clinic pleasant in many ways."[50] Diggs was preoccupied with his work and professional affiliations, but it fell to Beatrice to register the children for school and to establish ties in the local community where she knew no one and had no friends. Soon after arriving in Cleveland, she became pregnant and gave birth to their fourth child, Margaret Miller Diggs. The house, with several acres, was located on a dirt road about sixteen miles from the clinic in an area with a tumbling creek, a small lake, and a nearby park. It was an altogether ideal situation that they preferred. They played baseball with neighbors in a nearby empty lot. But there was only one family car, which Diggs used to go to work. At a butcher's shop where she purchased their meat, the owner and other customers were all from other countries and spoke languages that she could not understand. Because of the distance from the clinic, she could not assist Diggs with his presentations and slide shows as she had always done before. The kids seemed to be thriving, but Beatrice found life difficult, so in 1946 they moved into a house in a residential community, Cleveland Heights, much closer to the clinic.

They put the best face on the situation through the spring and summer, but it was already clear by August of 1947 that staying in Cleveland was no longer a viable option for the family. By this time, he was already making arrangements to return to Memphis. Beatrice returned to Memphis to find a home for them, which she found in the form of an antebellum house with seventeen acres in Cordova, Tennessee. He wrote to Ann, asking her to make sure to order the new equipment that he requested for the Gaston laboratory. He had submitted his resignation, and his last day would be at the end of the month. He still wanted to tie up all of the loose ends in Cleveland, so he would not be able to leave until sometime after that. Since they did not have a place to live in Memphis, he thought it would be necessary to leave the family in Cleveland until he could return to Memphis to find one. "Will be glad to be getting South and into teaching again," he wrote.[51] He would later recall, "I missed the South, [and] association with medical students and student technologists. I had rather be dead than live in industrial Cleveland the rest of my life."[52] With his usual optimism he looked forward to building up a real department in Memphis despite the burdensome teaching load. The Cleveland phase of his career was good not only for the experience that he acquired, but it also allowed for his absence from Memphis to be felt. Diggs was indeed missed, and he returned to Memphis with a full professorship and the commensurate boost in salary. "Opportunities were available at the time to be Dean at the University of Oklahoma and to be Director of Clinical Laboratories at the U. of Texas but I elected to go back to the University of Tennessee as Professor of Medicine in the Department of Clinical Pathology."[53]

Three months after moving into their antebellum home, it burned down, causing the family to be displaced. Fortunately no one was hurt, and they were not caught completely unprepared. While still living in Cleveland Heights, Diggs had made plans for a new house to be built there, which didn't happen due to the decision to return to Memphis. So, with some adaptations, the plans were used to build a shingled structure in Memphis.

The return was warm both in climate and in friendship. Diggs was glad to return to a laboratory with dedicated personnel and his work on sickle cell anemia, which had been absent during the war years and the time at the Cleveland Clinic. Ann Bell was showing great promise as a technical assistant, and Juanita Bibb, hired in 1940, had been directing the blood bank in Diggs's absence. Upon his return he resumed teaching the course in clinical laboratories, supervising the laboratories and the blood bank of the City of Memphis hospitals, and teaching students and residents. The children were growing. The oldest, Walter, was approaching high school, and Alice and John were respectively two and four years behind him. The youngest, Margaret, was thriving. Diggs looked forward to his work, at enjoying family life, and at finding a suitable home, preferably one in the country where he could grow a garden.

Although Diggs had not published on sickle cell anemia during this period, his interest in the disease continued. He saw patients when he could and interacted with colleagues. While still in Cleveland, he had an opportunity to spend some time in Washington, DC, at the Armed Forces Institute of Pathology. A former assistant from Diggs's laboratory in Memphis, Colin F. Vorder Bruegge, had risen to the rank of brigadier general and invited Diggs to examine the accessioned sickle cell cases there. As Diggs noted, "This led to my appointment as a Consultant in Pathology at the AFIP,"[54] which continued for many years. The experience also widened the circle of colleagues that he knew in his field.

To his surprise, the campus culture was different. It was evident that the influx of resources during and after the war years had changed everyone's sense of mission. The need for research was emphasized by these changes, and by accreditation reviews of the Medical Units, which called for an improvement in the amount of research. In response, Dr. Hyman made personnel changes that would encourage faculty to do more research, especially in the basic sciences. This came at a time after the war when faculty numbers increased and patient and teaching loads correspondingly decreased to more manageable levels. The war had galvanized a new, can-do spirit on campus that gave research a higher value.

Other aspects of city life around the campus did not change so quickly. The campus was located in a part of town that contained areas of poor black people, and a bayou ran along a street near the Baptist Hospital. The contrast was stark, as one newly arrived physician in 1942 noted: "Along the street was an open ditch and bordering this ditch were four or five structures, the backsides of which extended over the ditch, supported on stilts. Negro families were in residence, along with dogs, goats, chickens and at least one pig. All this looked strange for a medical center, and thought I must have lost my way; but the multistoried brick structure on my right turned out to be the south side of the Baptist Hospital."[55] He was newly arrived from California and in need of a house for himself and his wife. A colleague was able to help him out by letting him stay in her mother's house until they found something suitable. Behind this house, there was a barn-like structure where an elderly black man lived with his daughter. He was advised that the man was "'my nigger,' meaning, as I later found out, that he was to do chores for me and I was 'to take care of him'—an arrangement I came to find rather complicated."[56]

But the awareness of black Memphians was changing due to the Great Depression, which forced so many out of their communities to look for work, and the Second World War, which raised awareness of freedom, democracy, and equality. During the war, black workers organized unions and resisted the stereotypes of black laborers and inequities in pay. E. H. Crump's control of the city and county had been unerring and undeniable.

However, by 1940, his organization was becoming ineffectual due to the incompetent leadership of those in Crump's organization and the growing resistance among black citizens.[57] The Gaston Hospital was as segregated as the rest of the city and not exempt from racial disturbances.[58]

This was a challenging time for Diggs, as for everyone in the city. Before the war he had treated black patients and educated them about sickle cell anemia. He continued to educate even after being told by his dean, "We don't teach them."[59] He had started the first blood bank in the South and ignored the policy of strict segregation of blood units. He had done so without stepping outside his role as a healthcare provider. In part this was an expression of his personality, but it also stemmed from the training he had received in medical school, where he was encouraged to "maximize his medical and scientific contributions and minimize involvement with nonmedical, nonscientific activities."[60]

Diggs had been assigned to continue teaching the clinical pathology course, and to pursue his interest in sickle cell and other diseases, but the war had overshadowed everything. Now the pressures of the war, the increased patient and teaching loads, began to recede, and the campus assumed some of its normal appearance. One big difference that must have pleased Diggs was the increased emphasis on research. He had bemoaned the lack of a research mentality on campus, but the criticism by accrediting bodies and the wartime emphasis on research had changed that. The chief administrative officer, O. W. Hyman, took the issue on and began emphasizing that new faculty hires had to be made with an eye to expanding research.

Even though the campus of the Medical Units was infused with new ideas, buildings, and resources, there were changes occurring in the city. Memphis had been dominated by the Democratic Party for decades under the control of a political organization developed and run by Edward Hull Crump. Crump had served as mayor from 1909 to 1916, when he was removed as mayor by the Tennessee state legislature for violating the state's prohibition laws, after which time he consolidated his power in the county, enough to also be a powerful influence in state politics as well. He also served as a member of the U.S. House of Representative from 1932 to 1938, but his controlling influence extended to his death in 1954. In a town with such a high percentage of black citizens, he was able to maintain his position as the city's "boss," in part by encouraging them to vote, as long as they voted Democratic. In return for their vote, Crump gave them access to city services, such as a day just for blacks at the municipal zoo and black-only parks. Crump is credited with creating and controlling a political machine that gave black and other constituencies a measure of power and participation in the city and county governments while, at the same time, it subordinated them to Crump's agenda. As Crump's control of the organization weakened in the early 1940s, black demands increased for more political recognition and more power.

Although Diggs's list of publications did not reflect his activity in sickle cell anemia, he nevertheless continued his interest. After his stay at the Cleveland Clinic, he resolved to build a better department, and he began to think about organizational ways to carry out research into the nature of the disease. He knew that it was found in every organ system. That had been the principle lesson he learned from patients with disappearing spleens. So he engaged colleagues in various specialties to review and comment on the disease's manifestations. In this way he could educate as well as raise awareness about the disease: "We thought that this was of interest to the . . . orthopedic doctors . . . because of the bone changes. They were interesting to the eye doctors because . . . they had blindness as one of the manifestations. They were particularly interesting [to] the neurosurgeons because of the brain lesions. The gastrointestinal people were interested in it. The radiologists, of course, had a big part to play."[61] And so did pediatricians, pulmonary function, and kidney specialists. He involved physicians from other specialties by bringing them in to show them what he was doing or by sending them tissue samples and asking for their evaluations. In this way he established a local network of colleagues that both helped educate others on the ways sickle cell could affect the body and helped him in his research. He was exploring organ-system medicine well before it became an educational mantra in the 1960s.[62]

At the same time that medical knowledge and healthcare were expanding, so was interest in a national plan to pay for it. There was a glimmer of hope that federal funding in the form of national health insurance might become available. Such a plan might have made more health services available to blacks as well as the poor and unemployed. Beginning in 1943, a bill that came to be known as the Wagner-Murray-Dingell Bill had been debated as a serious amendment to the Social Security Act to provide payment, and thus medical care, for millions of uninsured and unemployed citizens. It would have included many black citizens. Opponents to the new bill branded it as "socialized medicine" and vilified the bill's proponents. Professional organizations that rejecting the bill included the American Medical Association, the American Nurses Associations, and the American Dental Association. The fear was that the bill would nationalize the healthcare professions, thus threatening to lower healthcare standards, eliminate the autonomy of providers, and destroy providers' relationships with patients. Key elements in the debate were the feeling of nationalism coming out of the war and the rising feeling of anti-communism that had an impact on all aspects of American life. Thus opponents were not reluctant to imply that proponents of the Wagner-Murray-Dingell Bill were themselves dupes of foreign, anti-American interests.[63]

Diggs debated in favor of the bill even as the AMA and other professional organizations vilified Wagner-Murray-Dingell as a subversive plot by foreign powers. He could see the debate was generating more heat than light, distracting attention from the real problem that the bill was intended to address, namely the millions of needy and uninsured people who were unable to take advantage of healthcare resources and who suffered needlessly. As a debater since his undergraduate days, he found himself in arguments with his colleagues about the bill and its implications. Diggs believed in making a thorough assessment of any issue before he made up his mind. This was true in politics, too, so when he voted on the issues, he tended to vote in support of the Democratic Party, while Beatrice tended to vote in favor of issues supported by the Republican Party. The Wagner-Murray-Dingell Bill was a product of the New Deal politics of Franklin Roosevelt, and was a progressive and liberal piece of legislation. When the war was won and confidence in the economy returned, however, political support shifted from the social planning and spending of the Democrats to the conservative and business-oriented Republicans, not to mention the escalating, acute fear of communism and the reactionary backlash of McCarthyism.

If Diggs had any concerns, it was not with how the benefits of national health insurance would affect patients, but how it might affect the political system. He believed in the individual responsibility of earning what you got, and the funding for the Wagner-Murray-Dingell plan would come from income taxes, so, in effect, people would be paying themselves for their healthcare. The worry for him was that people could come to expect that they had a natural right to healthcare, that healthcare should always be available. "It is the concept of something for nothing, of getting and not having put, which is dangerous. The shift of the responsibility from the individual and family or small social group to a large organization in which individual responsibility is lost is biologically wrong and will not work except in heaven where blood is not needed."[64] Diggs would continue to have this conversation as the national healthcare debate extended into the future.

Ever since 1910, when sickle cell was first identified, the disease was treated as a clinical entity characterized by skin ulcers and scars, enlarged glands, the yellow tinge of the sclera, and the "large number of thin, elongated, sickle-shaped and crescent-shaped forms" in the blood.[65] By the time Diggs joined the community of sickle cell researchers, the disease had moved from the clinic to the laboratory, where the correlation between the blood picture and patients' symptoms was of prime interest. For Diggs any attempt to understand the disease was closely linked to the patients who suffered from it. He needed to solve the problem of maintaining regular access to them in order to follow their progress. However, from the time the disease was identified to the late 1940s and beyond, it remained invisible to all but the scientists investigating it. Diggs's patients usually knew they had the disease only when he told them, which meant that, as a healer, he would be their sole source of information on how to control the disease in their individual lives.[66]

For many, the difficulties of the Great Depression seemed to evaporate with the onset of World War II, and the war seemed to open up the prospect of new opportunities in American life that would be unlike anything before. Diggs was ready to try something new and better. His older son observed: "He has always sought the truth and demanded good patient care—some might even call him a patient advocate."[67] This was true of his medical philosophy up to war's end but would also be a guiding principle during the postwar boom. On his return to Memphis from the Cleveland Clinic, Diggs wanted to build a better department. As the postwar years saw a dramatic increase in federal allocations for science, Diggs saw an opportunity to acquire the funding that up to now had remained elusive. Finally he would be able to translate his research interests into organizational structures that, he hoped, would better achieve his goals of better understanding of the disease and better patient care.

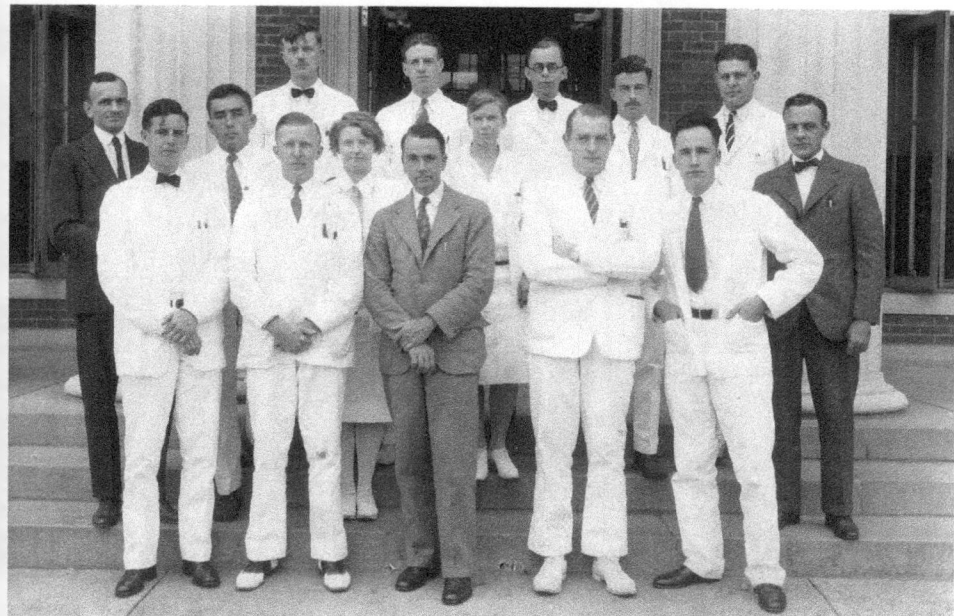

Diggs's University of Rochester class of 1927. Diggs is in the back row, third from the right.

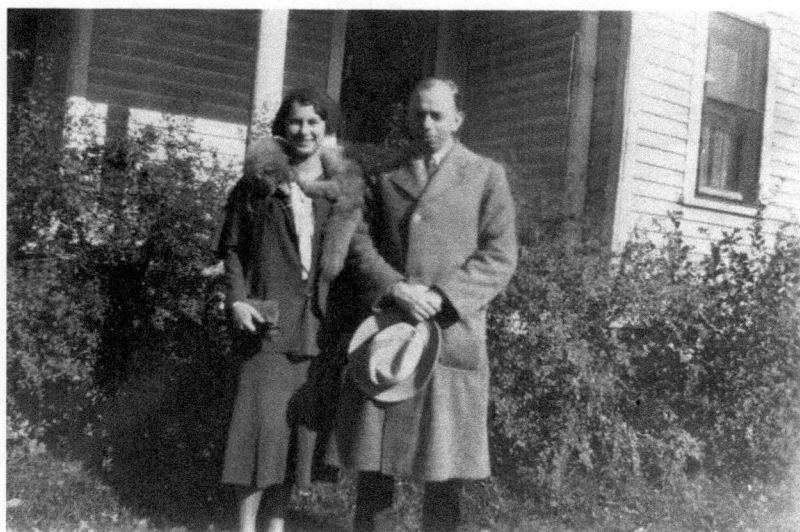

Whitley and Beatrice Diggs on their honeymoon in 1930.

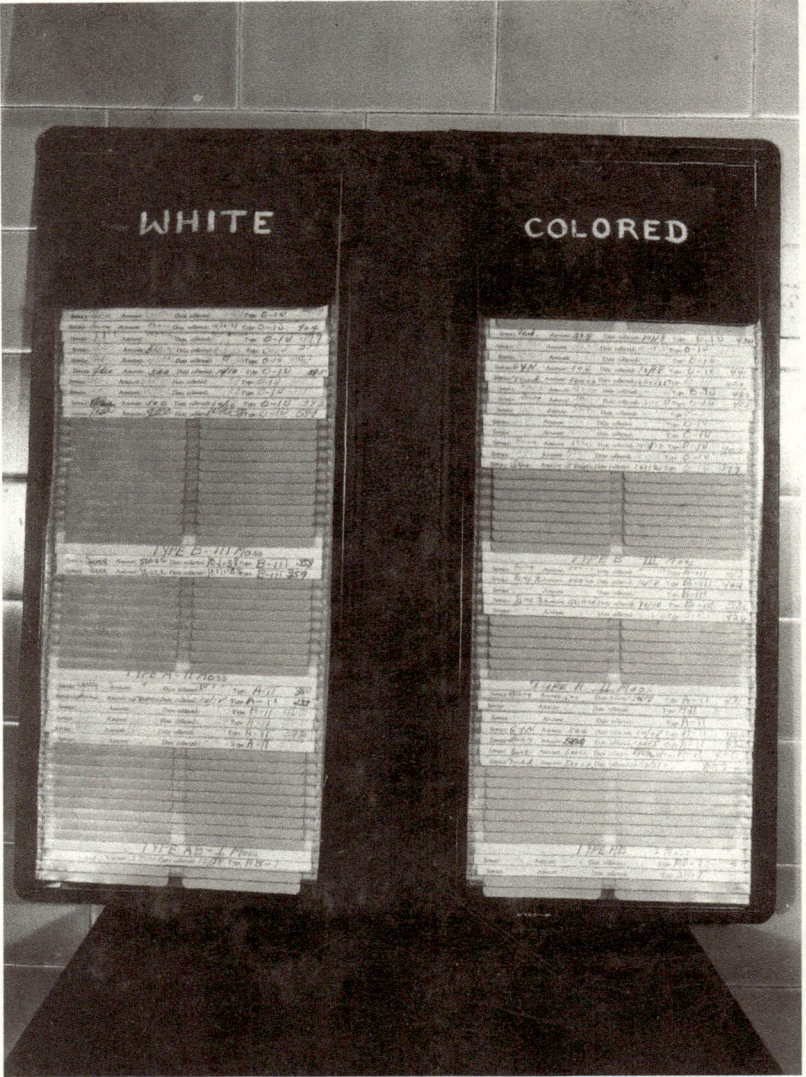

The file system used in 1938 in the John Gaston Hospital blood bank to record available blood units by race.

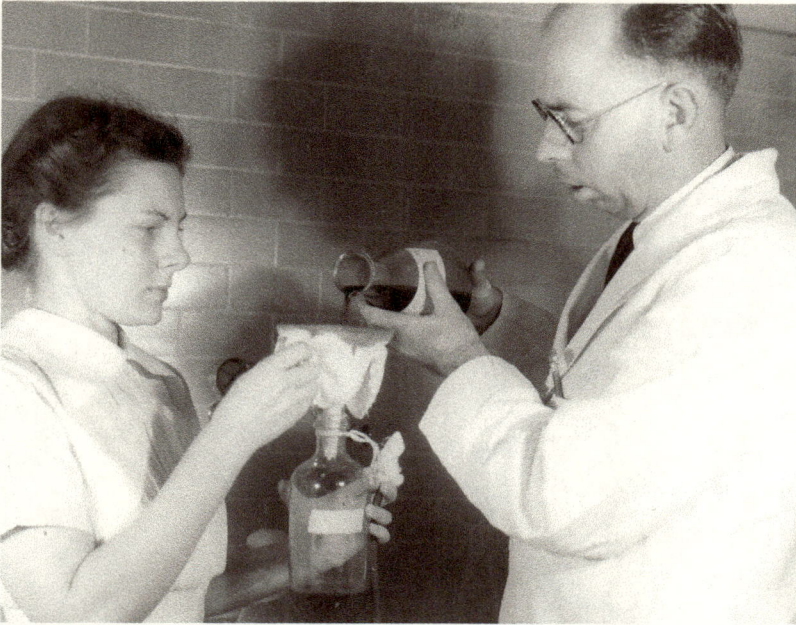

Nurse Alice Jean Keith holds the bottle and funnel while Diggs filters a unit of blood through sixteen layers of gauze. Notice the blood over the edge. Contamination quickly ensued, and the practice was replaced by a closed system.

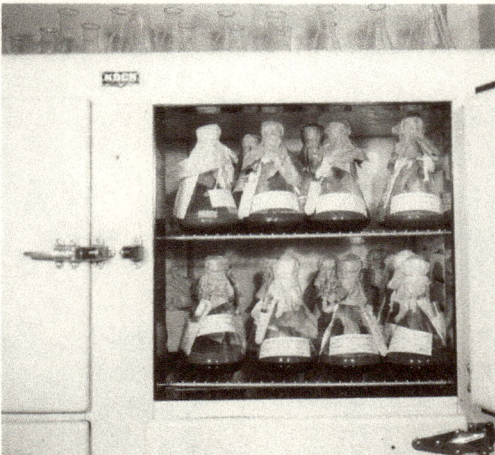

Blood units were initially stored in the refrigerator in Erlenmeyer flasks. As the blood bank's popularity increased, these flasks were replaced with milk bottles. Although the staff was expected to segregate the units within the refrigerator, enlargement of this image indicates that this was not done.

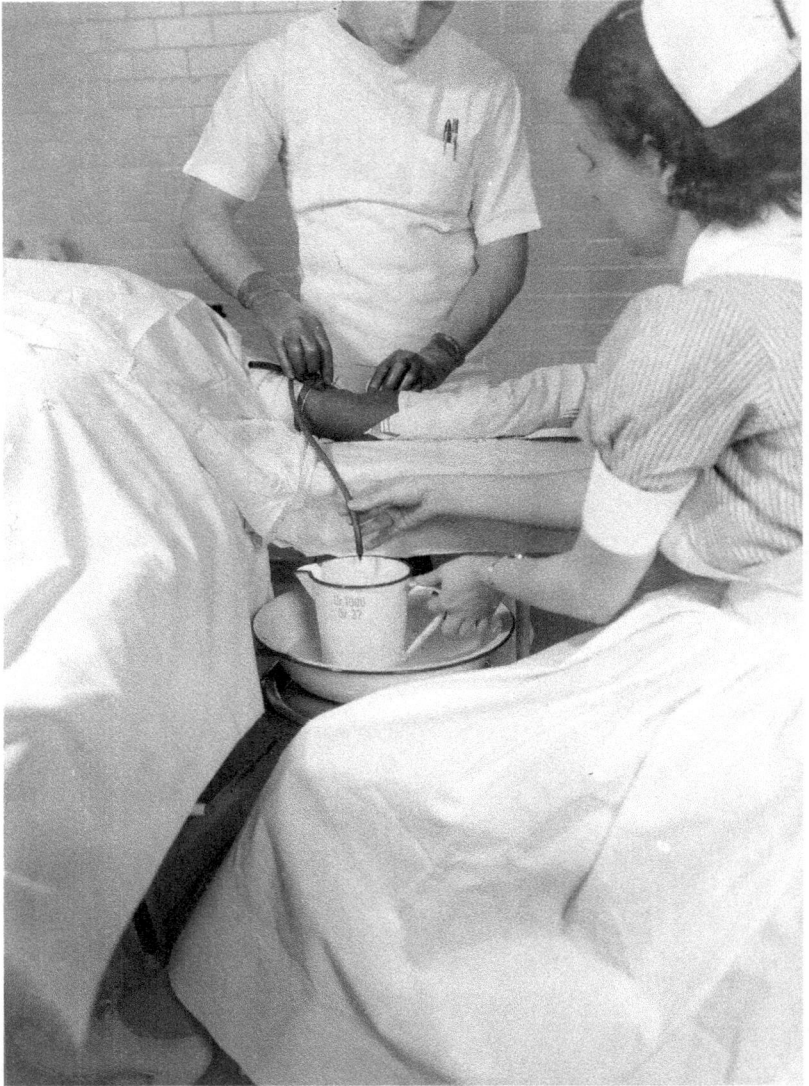

This is how blood was drawn in the initial days of the blood bank. Notice the needle placement ("meeting the blood head on") and the tube directing blood into an open container that is placed in a bowl of warm water to prevent clumping.

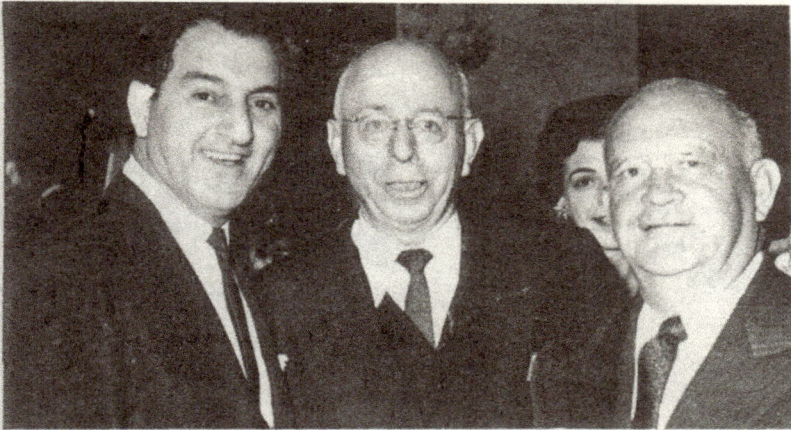

THE BIG THREE - Danny Thomas, Dr. Diggs and Edward Barry

Dr. Diggs together with entertainer and founder of St. Jude Children's Research Hospital Danny Thomas and fundraiser Edward Barry.

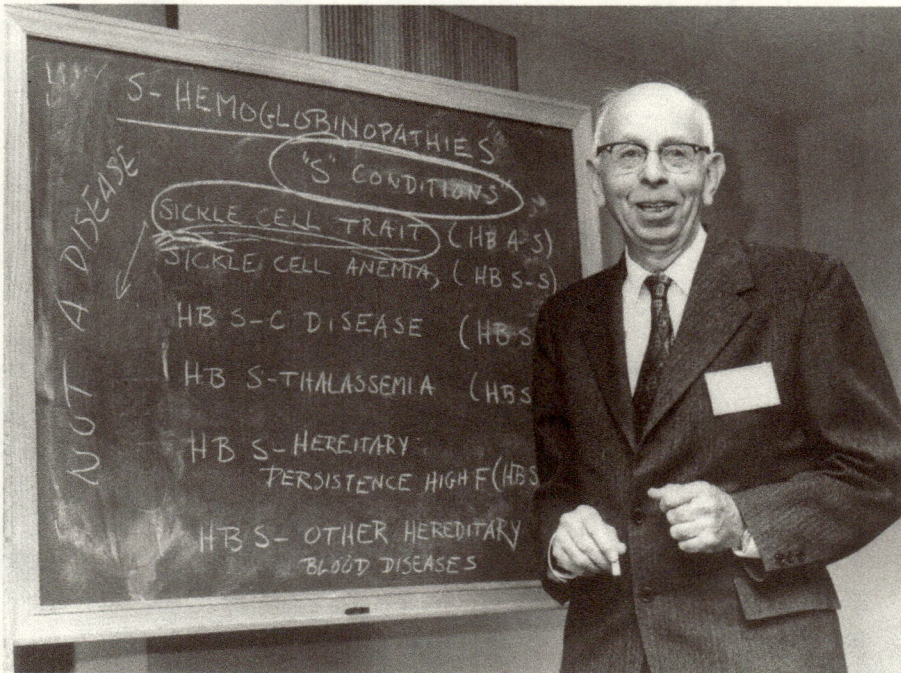

Diggs after a lecture at a technicians' meeting on sickle cell anemia given in Arkansas in 1973.

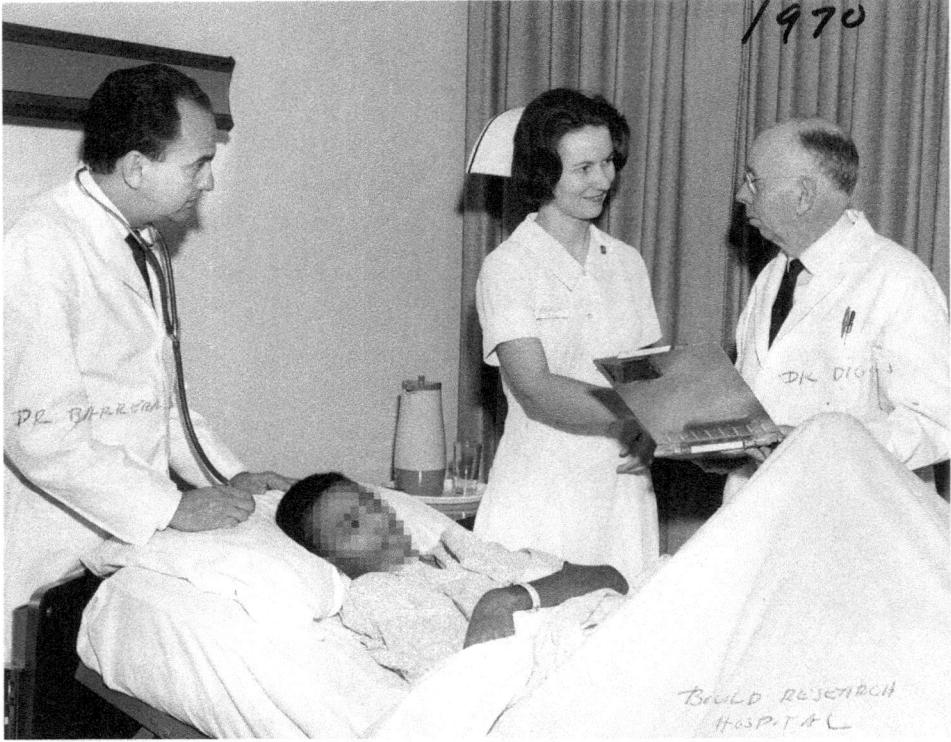

Dr. Diggs with a sickle cell patient. With him are Dr. Luis Barreras and Nurse Mary Dinkins.

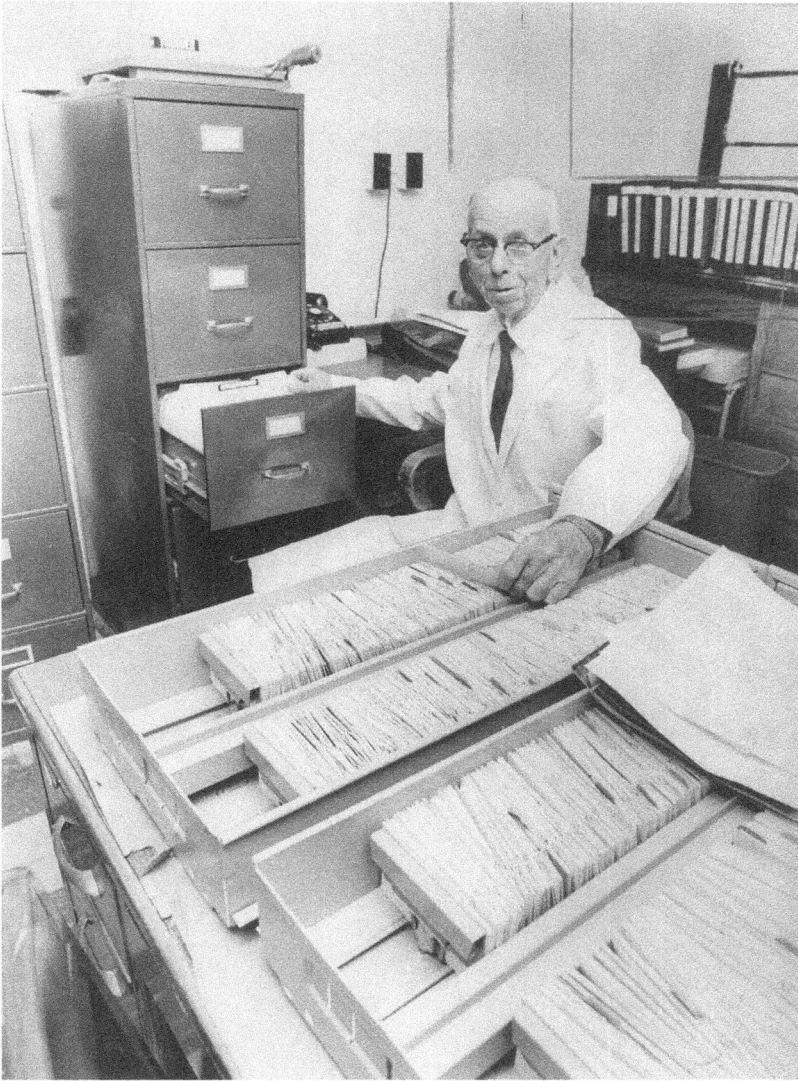

Diggs in 1976 after retirement, organizing his extensive data system on sickle cell patients.

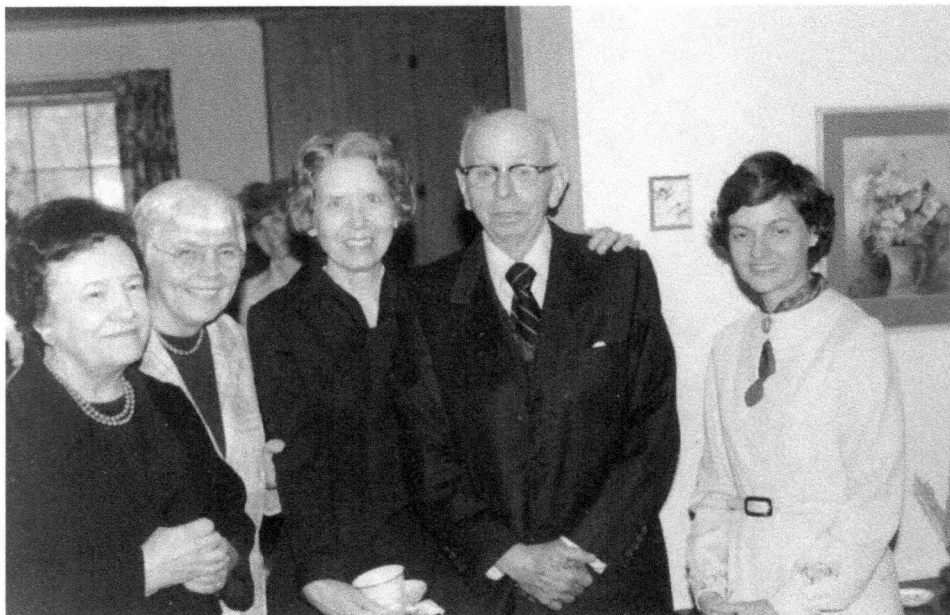

Probably around the time of his retirement, Diggs is seen here with (*left to right*) Jeanette Spann, Dr. Alys H. Lipscomb, Ann Bell, and Dr. Marion Dugdale.

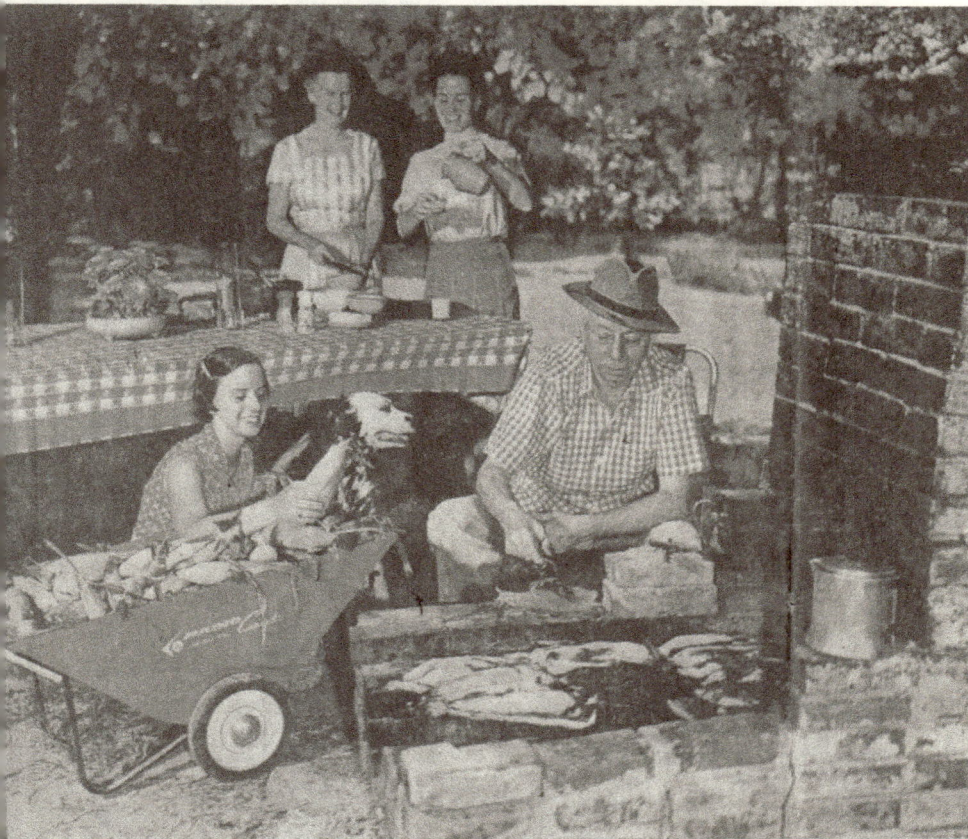

The L. W. Diggs Family Prepares Roasted Corn, Piece De Resistance, For Sunday Breakfast Guests
Peggy Helps Her Father, Dr. Diggs, While Mrs. Diggs and Daughter, Mrs. Charles Sullivan III, Make Ready the Table

A family picnic as recorded in the local newspaper.
Diggs is roasting homegrown corn.

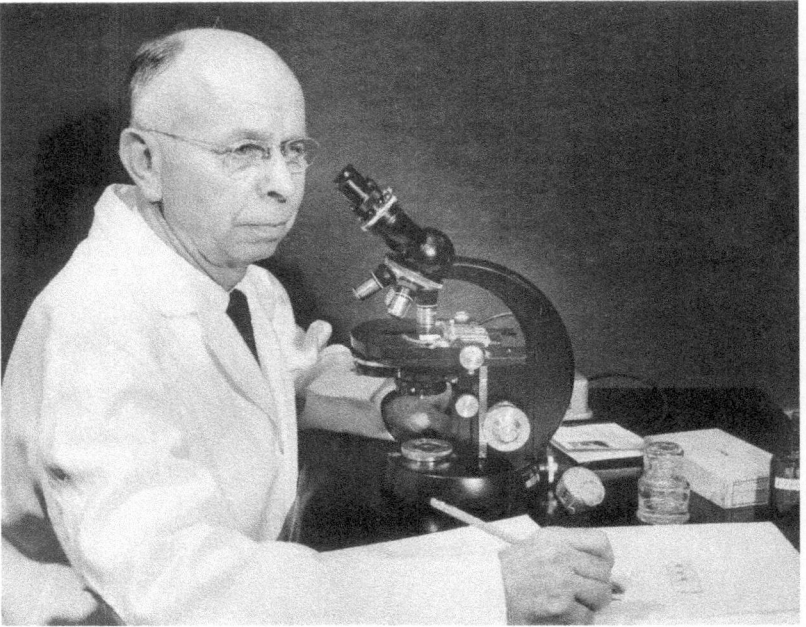

Diggs at his familiar place in front of a microscope.

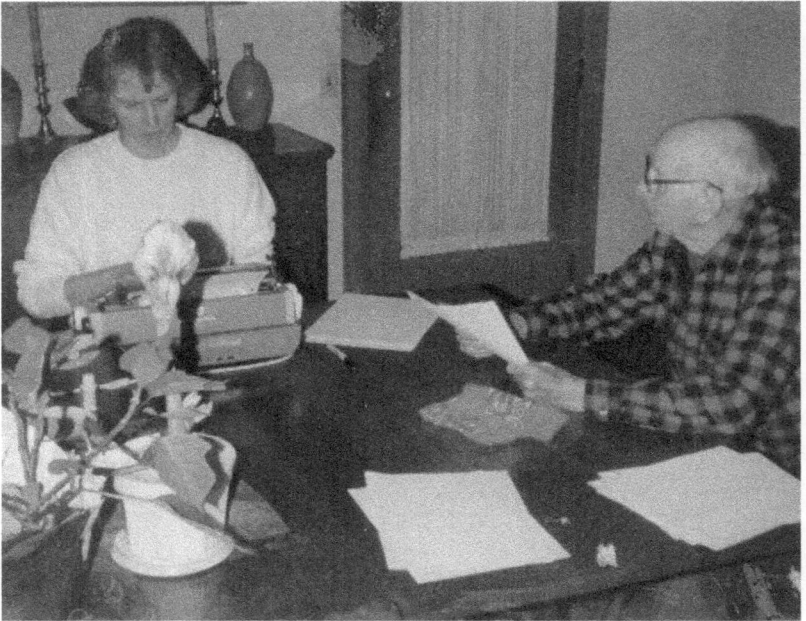

Diggs working on a letter to Hillary Clinton regarding
healthcare reform in the early 1990s.

A job half done is not done at all.
—My Daddy

Chapter 5
St. Jude and the Sickle Cell Center

Despite the opportunities and distractions of the war, Diggs returned to Memphis with a renewed dedication to his work and with plans to find better ways to address sickle cell anemia. He had been carrying out sickle cell research since he had arrived in Memphis in 1929, and had conducted it largely without assistance before the war. He had worked to accumulate a group of patients that trusted him and whom he could see with a regularity that would let him plot a picture of sickle cell's patterns. And he had involved colleagues in the evaluation of patients with interesting symptoms or findings related to their specialties. He was finding ways to overcome the invisibility of the disease, thus increasing his activity in the areas that interested him the most: research, along with treating and educating patients. As the focus of the nation in the late 1940s and early 1950s shifted from winning the devastating war in Europe and Asia to the Cold War, the booming economy, and a swelling civil rights movement, there was now substantial growth in the federal research dollars to support seemingly every kind of scientific research, though still not for sickle cell research.

Diggs began devising new ways to better understanding the disease that would both have practical value for his patients and enable him to build a "real department."[1] He had advanced as far as he could at the UT Medical Units. He participated in conferences, published papers and book chapters, communicated with everyone he could identify in his field, and he knew as much as anyone did about the disease. Although he was a researcher as well as a clinician, his major concern was always for maximizing the health of his patients. As the majority of sickle cell researchers moved into the more theoretical area of molecular biology, Diggs began to feel that an organizational solution would serve his needs far better, a framework that would capitalize on the work already done with the group of patients he was able to assemble and the community of researchers. Such a solution would ideally facilitate a regular discourse between patients and researchers for the benefit of the patients.

As part of his early interest in what was known and the range of ineffective therapies, Diggs gathered publications on the treatment of the disease, which he summarized and supplemented with his own observations. In essence, he could only conclude that too little was known: "There is a dearth of information concerning the natural course of sickle-cell anemia in all its varied manifestations, and the possibility of spontaneous remissions must be considered in the evaluation of favorable therapeutic responses. The effectiveness of any form of therapy in the treatment of sickle-cell anemia remains to be proved."[2] Little would change in the years since he made that statement. The most striking feature of the disease was its ability to cause patients to cry out in excruciating pain. Diggs avoided using the strongest remedies available—opiates and their derivatives—because they suppressed respiration and thereby oxygen for the body, something that could trigger or exacerbate a crisis; and because of the likelihood of addiction, which would make a patient's life worse rather than better, and because these drugs were not strong enough to manage the worst pain. Finding a way to decipher the mystery of this disease would preoccupy Diggs for the remainder of his life.

Part of the reason why his research in sickle cell subsided at this time was connected with the war. From the late 1930s to 1949, very little new research was being conducted. Little progress was being made in creating new knowledge about the disease and, despite the research completed to date, nothing new had emerged therapeutically that would relieve the symptoms. Without more knowledge, researchers could do little more than repeat what had already been done.[3] The discovery that would again change the face of sickle cell research and increase understanding of the underlying mechanism of the disease came in 1949 with a publication by Linus Pauling and Harvey Itano showing that the sickling effect in red cells was due to a defect that had been located in the globin portion of the hemoglobin molecule.[4] The work by Pauling and Itano exemplified the kind of pure research that Diggs chose not to pursue. Studying the disease separately from the illness was foreign to his way of thinking. Although the discovery by Pauling and Itano was of promising importance, it was an abstract achievement separated from Diggs's preferred proximity to the patient. He remained interested in exploring the clinicopathological features of the disease in the hope that some finding would lead to an amelioration if not an outright cure. Nevertheless, all research was important to him because a breakthrough could come from anywhere.

After Diggs returned from the Cleveland Clinic, his research focused on a deeper analysis of the ways in which sickle cell manifests in all parts of the body. The mechanism of the disease was becoming familiar. Once the cells sickled, red cells lost the spongy quality that allowed them to navigate through capillaries that were often smaller in diameter than the red cells themselves. When they assumed their familiar grotesque and pointed shape, sickled cells were rigid and could aggregate to form occlusions or blockages that prevented further blood flow through the vessels. At this point the damage would be compounded because, as the blood flow slowed and then ceased, the available oxygen would further decrease, causing the damaged areas to increase gradually. Since an occlusion could happen anywhere in the body, the disease was also known as a masquerader that, without competent testing, could be misdiagnosed as other diseases, such as arthritis or pneumonia.[5] Finding a way to intervene was crucial to Diggs's goals as a researcher and a clinician. With this in mind, he considered how best to realize his concept of a clinical center by applying what he had learned from his experiences in designing and organizing the Gaston Hospital and the Cleveland Clinic Blood Bank.

While he was forming his ideas, another, related opportunity became available to him and the university. After 1955, Diggs gained additional organizing experience by becoming active as a member on a citywide steering committee to help Danny Thomas locate and build a new pediatric hospital in Memphis, which would be an experience in creating a new kind of hospital. The project would later become the St. Jude Children's Research Hospital, which would work in tandem with Diggs's own Sickle Cell Center to create a greater awareness of sickle cell and other blood disease in the Memphis area.

Diggs drew on all of this experience, plus the funding from various new and old sources, to create a sickle cell center. He continued to build a better program by finding ways to educate his profession on the multiple manifestations of sickle cell. As he was planning he also continued his efforts to promote the value of clinical pathology to the medical community. Together with his wife, Beatrice, and Ann Bell, he conducted hundreds of workshops for pathologists and technologists in various parts of the country. He developed a fascination for finding ways to use photographic technology to illustrate what he had learned about the morphology of blood cells, which complimented the importance he placed on hand-drawn anatomical illustration. Since his student days he had been interested in studying the forms that blood cells took in health and disease and in showing how they appeared at the different stages of their development. He began looking for a way to create realistic, high-quality images in the tradition of Max Brödel, his medical illustration instructor at Hopkins, and Joseph L. Scianni in the Pathology Department.

At some point soon after the war, Diggs made the acquaintance of a Memphis artist by the name of Dorothy Sturm, who had a national reputation for her watercolors and enamels. She also had an interest in medical illustration. Diggs understood the value of being able to draw what he observed, and he often included his illustrations in his publications. His daughter Alice likewise became interested in drawing, and she would contribute many drawings to his workshops and publications over the years.[6] What intrigued him about Sturm was the prospect of making definitive images for teaching that would incorporate everything that was known at the time about the appearance of the cells. With the help of Ann Bell, Sturm set up a microscope in her home to use for the observations that she would include in her drawings. She produced fifty-seven watercolors that depicted blood cells in various forms, including erythrocytes, granulocytes, plasmocytes, monocytes, and neutrophils, along with a series on infectious mononucleosis. The unique combinations of shapes, colors, and textures revealed by the microscope fascinated her. She had established her reputation at a time when there was an increasing demand for the illustrator's talents, and few were adept at communicating visually what could be seen through a microscope.[7]

Sturm's images were idealized in the sense that they were based on everything that was known about blood cells at the time and illustrated what the viewer should see through a microscope without the interference or confusion of adjacent structures and artifacts that could be found in blood smears. Diggs commissioned these images from her for use as a teaching aid for faculty and students, and for years they hung on the walls of the Department of Clinical Pathology for anyone to study and review.[8] This collaboration with Sturm was so successful that Diggs further commissioned her to produce images for a book he was working on that would cover the topic completely. In 1954, his classic *The Morphology of Blood Cells* was published, and would prove to be his most enduring book-length work.[9] He shared the credit with Sturm and Bell by making them coauthors, an act that illustrated his generosity, humility, and collaborative spirit.

Although Diggs was not outspoken about health-insurance reform, he saw a need for it in the patients he treated. He was aware that the biggest obstacle to access to medicine was cost. Although the movement to reform the way healthcare was funded began haltingly in FDR's administration during the Depression years, it failed to attract sufficient congressional support for passage. In President Truman's administration, healthcare and civil rights became domestic priorities. The 1943 Wagner-Murray-Dingell Bill inspired a public relations battle between the medical communities led by the American Medical Association and the U.S. Public Health Service. The American Medical Association pooled large amounts of money and support to fund the largest public relations campaign that anyone had seen for the purpose of defeating universal health insurance. The AMA characterized Wagner-Murray-Dingell as an extension of the communist design on world domination, an attack on the doctor-patient relationship, and an attempt to subordinate doctors to the federal bureaucracy. Diggs welcomed the federal government's move to expand Social Security to include basic health insurance for everyone. In this way, he was in opposition to the majority of his colleagues and most professional organizations, but he did not participate directly in the national debate.

The debate between the federal government and the medical community was vitriolic at times. It often ignored the facts and seldom focusing on those who would have benefited from access to the healthcare system. The bill remained for consideration in Congress for ten years before its supporters abandoned it.[10] Diggs knew as well as anyone could that insurance made a significant difference in healthcare. He was well aware that many of his patients often delayed seeing a doctor because of the cost until their illness forced them to seek help, which meant that illnesses, such as those often seen at public hospitals like Gaston, were advanced and complicated, and much more expensive to treat than they would have been if treated earlier. At the same time, however, he did not believe that anyone had a right or entitlement to healthcare paid for by others, but rather that health was an obligation of the individual. Basing the health insurance reform on a wage tax to pay for medical care would have appealed to him. The concept of something for nothing was unacceptable to him and a corrupting influence on society. If government were to assist, then it should be the local and not the federal government that should participate. A local government would be more sensitive to the concerns that were specific to the community and more responsive to the electorate that it served. And there were others who speculated that his support of the bill led to his being scrutinized by the Federal Bureau of Investigation. He was not investigated, as it turned out, but the paranoid feelings of anti-communism and the Cold War were pervasive.[11]

Diggs continued attending conferences; workshops, which had begun during the war; and clinical pathology and medical technology seminars. He spoke on the issues that concerned him, and would include American historical sources that were close to him. One admirer wrote him: "It was people like you who signed the Declaration of Independence."[12] Diggs's view was derived in part from his understanding of what rights were from George Mason and the Virginia Declaration of Rights of 1776 as well as the history of that document.[13] He also gave lectures when invited to do so. His style was straightforward and easy to follow. At a typical presentation on the morphology of blood cells given to a group of medical technology students, he would present each cell and discuss its appearance under the microscope, leavening the presentation with humor—such as referring to an unfamiliar cell as "What the cell is that?"[14] Beatrice very often accompanied him on these trips to assist him during presentations; she also acted as his typist and editor. Often, too, Ann Bell accompanied them when they traveled.

With his teaching, clinical, service, and outreach activities, Diggs's workload was considerable. He still directed the blood bank as well. On one occasion he must have appeared overloaded to the blood bank staff, for they created a drawing to cheer him up. It acknowledged that "things have been tough for you lately"[15] and recommended that he "let up a bit. You are working too hard. Let the G.P [general pathology] lab, and the House Staff lab, go to pot one day. Chances are that the next day the problems will have smoothed out or better still you may have thought of a way to smooth them. All of this probably does not make sense, but at least we are not asking for anything."[16] Diggs took the time to write letters to local media regarding the creation of a large park that would preserve a pastoral setting in the Memphis area. He argued against the "jingle of money created by new payrolls, the noise of factories, of heavy trucks and shifting freight cars,"[17] and in favor of a park with golf courses, restricted areas for horseback riding, polo and rodeos, and fishing and picnicking.

Applying himself completely to whatever he did was Diggs's normal way of conducting himself. He pursued his scientific interests but also dedicated himself to the mentoring of colleagues. In this context, his colleagues remember him well. In honor of his sixtieth birthday, they pooled their resources to hire a local artist, Billy Price Hosmer, to paint a life-size portrait of Diggs. The portrait itself was vintage Diggs, as seen through the eyes of family, friends, and colleagues. In it he was seated at a laboratory bench, resting his elbow on the surface only a few inches away from a binocular, oil-immersion microscope, with his right hand resting on his knee and holding a pencil. His expression is of someone preparing to tell a humorous story or communicate an interesting finding. The group to honor Diggs met on May 28, 1961. Fred Kraus introduced those present, including the artist; the College of Medicine dean, Maston Callison; Lorraine Kraus; Ann Bell; Lou and Henry Packer; and Jimmy Hughes. Beatrice was there with their daughters, Alice and Peggy. The main speaker, Alys Lipscomb, spoke about what Diggs meant to her personally and to many others on campus. "We are agreed," she began, "that the impact of his character is imprinted sharply where it will do the most good—in the minds of his students and associates."[18] The portrait is a reminder of the man they all knew and loved for his kindness and wit. Lipscomb told those attending that the artist had captured "the informality of [his] typical pose, the twinkle in the eye, which bespeaks his tremendous sense of humor."[19] The effect that Diggs's personality and style had on his students could not be captured in his familiar features in the portrait. Lipscomb pointed out that he would be remembered "locally, nationally, and internationally not only for his brilliant research in the field of hematology in general and sickle cell anemia in particular, but also for his "down home" farmer-type analogies which students so dearly love."[20] Included in his analogies was a description of the eosinophilic granulocyte as "round, regular, sharply refractile and fall[ing] off the nucleus like a sack of potatoes would fall off a mule's back."[21]

Diggs taught medical students, but also nursing and medical technology students: "he taught them vocabulary, prefixes, suffixes and how to put them together. Testing his skill and their knowledge, he asked them a list of definitions once. Amongst the words included was 'laminectomy.' One of the logical answers was 'A Caesarian section on a sheep.'" Lipscomb started her professional career as a medical technologist. However, with Diggs's encouragement and support, she pursued her medical degree and enjoyed a long and successful career at the University of Tennessee. Along with a copy of her presentation remarks to Diggs for his files, she included a postscript: "You'll never know how important you have been in my life. You've always been there when I needed help. You gave me my first job. You showed me I could teach. You encouraged me to go to medical school. You introduced me to Dr. Haden, paving the way to my internship and fellowship. You gave me my second job. You have championed my cause through 50 years. The help you've given me is similar to the help you've given so many."[22] This presentation was made when Diggs was sixty-one years old. Along with the commemoration of his retirement, the university named him Goodman Professor of Medicine in 1968, and professor emeritus in medicine-hematology in 1969.[23]

In 1955, Memphis mayor Frank Tobey received a query from Danny Thomas about constructing a hospital for underprivileged children. Thomas had been advised by a friend, Archbishop of Chicago Samuel Cardinal Stritch, to build it in Memphis because the cardinal had started his career in Memphis and considered it his hometown. Thomas sent an advisor, who was welcomed enthusiastically by city representatives, including Mayor Frank T. Tobey, who had a special interest in children's issues since his wife had suffered a miscarriage. Tobey promised the support of the city, which included donating the land for the hospital. In response, Thomas invited Tobey and his advisors to Hollywood for further discussions. With so many positive developments, Tobey returned to Memphis, where he informed the medical and other city leaders of the prospect of such a hospital. By May, Thomas himself was in Memphis, talking to people and fundraising for the new hospital. The bond between Tobey and Thomas grew quickly in a short time. When Tobey succumbed unexpectedly to a severe heart attack in September, Thomas was deeply affected.[24]

Even though the mayor and some leading Memphians welcomed the idea of a new hospital, not everyone in the medical community liked the idea. One objection came from those who felt that Memphis already had a strong medical center for pediatric diseases. The Le Bonheur Children's Hospital had already been built and, after Tobey's death, an addition was built to the Memphis City Hospital, the Frank T. Tobey Memorial Children's Hospital. In addition, the private hospitals in the city also had beds set aside for pediatric patients. In 1955, O. W. Hyman, then chief executive officer of the University of Tennessee Medical Units, saw a possible solution: "[If] patients admitted to the hospital are limited to those with certain diseases or groups of diseases, and if the hospital is so equipped as to provide special facilities for the specially skilled staff, then the hospital will serve a much wider area and will in addition provide treatment opportunities not otherwise made available by local community institutions."[25]

Hyman did not offer a way to make this plan financially viable, but he was already moving the thinking in a more specialized direction. The worry was that St. Jude would compete with Le Bonheur and the other existing hospitals, in effect reducing the number of patients for them and thus reducing the teaching opportunities for medical students. It would also be a hardship on families traveling long distances, who would have to afford room and board during long stays. Another difficulty seen by doctors, including Diggs, went to the heart of Thomas's desire to build a hospital with national prominence that was open to everyone. Thomas wanted a facility with an international calling. However, the difficulty was that a hospital treating all childhood diseases might be forced to limit itself to the local population and to treating only their diseases.[26]

Diggs had been a part of the plans for St. Jude from their inception. He and James N. Etteldorf from the Department of Pediatrics were supposed to monitor Danny Thomas as part of their activities, and to keep their UT colleagues informed. It was probably the case for members on both sides of the negotiation to keep their respective leaderships informed about key planning developments and to identify key details that might tip the scales in favor of one side or the other. When Thomas learned about the monitors, he had Diggs appointed to represent the Memphis and Shelby County Medical Society as a member of the St. Jude Steering Committee along with Etteldorf, a veteran pediatrician who started the pediatrics program at the university, to represent the University of Tennessee. Ed Barry, a well-respected Memphis fundraiser noted for his work on behalf of Baptist Hospital and Methodist Hospital, chaired the steering committee. Its task was to turn Danny Thomas's dream into a reality: to create a world-class hospital that would help underserved and underprivileged children with leukemia. Thomas and the committee came to rely on Diggs's knowledge of childhood blood illnesses, such as sickle cell, hemophilia, and leukemia, as well as his straightforward and clear approach to solving problems.

In the first year or so, Diggs solved the problem of what kind of hospital St. Jude would be by suggesting to the steering committee a focus on the hematology and oncology of childhood diseases.[27] According to J. V. Simone, "Diggs advised Thomas and the trustees to change the plans and build a research facility for the study and treatment of blood diseases and cancer in children; they accepted his recommendation."[28] Diggs always saw patient care and research as interwoven, and his participation on the steering committee was crucial. His ideas appealed to Thomas and the committee so much that they adopted them as the central direction for the new hospital. As Hazel Fath reported, "With this decision, the picture changed. The medical community and the staff at the medical school recognized the potential involved in the creation of a national research center. They noted that it would stimulate training in both research and clinical studies."[29] The advantage for the local hospitals was that beds for long-term study would be at St. Jude, while beds for acute, short-term, and curable patients would be located at the local hospitals. In order for the new hospital to be open to any child, funding would come from donations and research grants; any child who fit into one of the research programs would be admitted to the hospital at no cost. As Diggs stated, "Since these diseases affect all races, all children will be admitted."[30] Staff members would be selected "who are best qualified regardless of race or creed."[31]

For St. Jude this meant that its patients could indeed come from national and even international locations. Thomas was grateful to Diggs for making the initial suggestion of a research hospital.[32]

St. Jude Thaddeus was the patron saint of hopeless causes. And perhaps it was Diggs's commitment to helping those afflicted with sickle cell anemia that drew him to Thomas. Within their relationship, Diggs formulated the idea that St. Jude could flourish as a hospital specializing in research into catastrophic diseases, which both set it apart from other hospitals and addressed a wider patient base. The concept also relieved concerns that St. Jude might compete with existing hospitals because it would not draw away the acute-care cases that the children's hospitals addressed, but at the same time, it would offer hope to those with difficult, chronic illnesses. Diggs's vision helped shape the direction of the hospital.[33]

There was excitement mixed with doubt at the idea of opening a new hospital in Memphis. Diggs was one of those who saw the project's potential, but he also had some understandable concerns. The St. Jude Children's Research Hospital was a bold initiative with few if any peers anywhere in the world. Diggs was unsure whether the project would evolve in the way the steering committee envisioned, given the uncertainties that had been voiced by his medical colleagues. Diggs was drawn to "Danny's Dream" and its potential for a new way to organize and practice medicine that had always been part of his thinking and that would provide a new venue in Memphis for sickle cell research.

Danny Thomas sponsored a number of well-publicized fundraising events in Memphis that included prominent Hollywood stars. At one such event in 1957, Diggs and his wife bought tickets to a fundraiser that was held in Russwood Park, the minor-league baseball stadium across the street from Baptist Hospital. He was reluctant to attend but felt a duty to do so. "It had been raining," he would tell a gathering of St. Jude supporters a few years later, "and there was a very black cloud in the west with occasional lightning flashes and rolling thunder. A bad storm and heavy rain seemed imminent. Soon after that the winds changed. The skies cleared. Instead of a black and threatening cloud there was a bright evening star right over the area where the St. Jude Hospital was being built."[34] Although the evening star was a naturally recurring event, he represented it to his audience as a sign that "the St. Jude cause was worthy and should be vigorously supported.[35]" This rhetorical flourish emphasized his unquestioning acceptance of St. Jude as a "bright evening star" and a turning point away from any remaining doubts that he had about the development of the hospital. His support of St. Jude solidified, and his participation in its growth and welfare would continue for the rest of his life.

Diggs also participated in the founding of St. Jude in other ways. He helped in the organizing of staffing duties and in the writing of policies that would govern the staff's activities. Along with Etteldorf and others, he participated in the search to find the first medical director for St. Jude. The national search identified a number of promising candidates before settling on Donald Pinkel, who was the hospital's first employee, hired while the building was still under construction in 1961.

Diggs's participation in St. Jude's creation was gratifying, but not without its headaches for him and for other members of the St. Jude and University of Tennessee communities. In 1960, Diggs was appointed to the St. Jude Board of Governors and the Board of Directors. From the beginning through the 1960s, almost everyone connected with St. Jude and the University of Tennessee Medical Units assumed that there would be close ties between the institutions. The addition of the St. Jude facility to the university's portfolio would be a welcome enhancement to the university's research stature. The researchers at St. Jude could also benefit from having faculty status and access to the broader range of research that was an essential part of a university. These expectations were unfulfilled, however, because from the mid-1950s onward much effort at both institutions had been expended on organizing and building St. Jude, but no formal affiliation agreement was concluded between the two institutions that defined what their relationship would be or how it would be formulated in policy. During 1960 and 1961, Diggs and the steering committee were busy with a national search for St. Jude's first physician-in-chief, and concomitantly the star-shaped hospital building was being constructed. Nevertheless, as the 1960s arrived, the new hospital's leadership felt increasingly independent and unwilling to accept a constraining relationship with an institution of lesser status.[36]

The feelings of participants on both sides hardened to the point that what had started as a crack between the two institutions grew into a deep divide. In 1969 there was genuine concern on the part of university planners that the divide would be permanent. Diggs may have been the only person who stood in the relative good graces of both sides. In April he called upon the St. Jude Board of Governors to have a meeting between St. Jude and the University of Tennessee—the result of which was the formation of a liaison committee. The St. Jude medical director, Donald Pinkel, was hopeful: "I hope through Dr. Diggs' good offices, we can get discussions of the University of Tennessee–St. Jude relationship back to the faculty level."[37] While Diggs was an acceptable intermediary on St. Jude's behalf, his role was not always viewed favorably by the university's negotiators. The chair of the Pediatrics Department, upon hearing that the university was expected to "deal through Dr. Diggs," reportedly told Diggs that "he would not deal through him to St. Jude, but only through the Dean and Chancellor."[38] Additionally, low-key talks took place between the two sides that produced no concrete results. Yet neither side could give up entirely on the relationship, so the talks continued. In December of 1971, almost ten years after the opening of St. Jude, a formal affiliation agreement was finally and painstakingly developed. Diggs's role was pivotal; his support was for both St. Jude and the university, but his position sometimes provoked harsh criticism from his colleagues.

Diggs undoubtedly saw St. Jude as an opportunity to participate in the creation of another research venue for sickle cell research, perhaps one that was better funded and organized. He had had experience in organizing and managing departments when he was a resident at the University of Rochester's newly built Strong Memorial Hospital and throughout his career at the University of Tennessee. He had organized their laboratories, and at the University of Tennessee Medical Units and the Cleveland Clinic he had organized blood banks. It made sense to him that, as resources became available, he would create another organization related to his central interest: a sickle cell center where all aspects of the disease—from the laboratory to the bedside to the home—could be given concentrated attention.

Whereas Diggs could foresee funding for St. Jude grounded in the appeal of catastrophic childhood illnesses, the same attraction would not hold true for a disease like sickle cell. The creation of the Sickle Cell Center and the funding for it happened more slowly and on a parallel path. At about the same time that work with the St. Jude Steering Committee was progressing, Diggs began creating the groundwork for a sickle cell clinic within the university's Gailor Clinic. Even though money was available for basic and clinical research, "Granting agencies," Diggs recalled, "considered [sickle cell] an unimportant disease involving blacks and not worthy of study."[39] However, beginning in 1953 the Herbert Herff Foundation donated ten thousand dollars to Diggs for basic research into sickle cell anemia and renewed it the following year.[40] Herff was the same Memphis philanthropist who had donated the initial funding for opening the blood bank in 1938.

The work on the Sickle Cell Center went forward, with rooms donated by the University of Tennessee for Diggs's use, so that in the following year the foundation renewed its support. The funding made it possible for Diggs to hire a technical assistant, James Childs, an African American phlebotomist in the Gailor Clinic "whose main duty was to provide transportation for patients in the community and to assist in blood collection and examination in order to obtain information about hematological and chemical changes in relation [to] the recurrent crises."[41] Years before, Childs had worked in the laboratory of Dr. Alfred Blalock at Vanderbilt University before moving to Johns Hopkins University Medical School. This was the same Blalock who bored a hole in Diggs's skull to relieve pressure on his brain after he bumped his head on a tree limb while still a medical student. The transportation employed by Childs was Diggs's car, which Childs used to bring patients without means to the clinic and take them home afterwards. This practice partially solved the problem of patients not keeping their appointments by addressing their chronic lack of funds for transportation. Having Childs transport them may also have allayed patients' potential fears of coming to the hospital. For Diggs to arrive at such a solution was extraordinary in the Jim Crow era and manifested his commitment to live by certain principles of fairness and compassion to all people, regardless of skin color. This also helped to provide a group of patients who could serve as a foundation for Diggs's research, patients he could follow regularly for longer periods of time.[42] The money for this work was administered by the university and announced by O. W. Hyman, the university's executive officer. Diggs preferred to let the university handle the money as a way of demonstrating that every penny was being used for the purpose for which it was given.

James Childs did more than transport patients. Before coming to Memphis, Child had received some medical training while working as a medical technologist in Alfred Blalock's laboratory at Vanderbilt University. With the training he received, he was in a good position to recognize the importance of sickle cell to the black community. "He was one of the first blacks to believe that sickle cell was an inherited disease and, based on [Diggs's] work, to educate the black community on that."[43] He had to convince African Americans that the disease existed. In a 1962 newspaper story, he was greatly inspired by the work in Memphis and felt "that too many Negroes both professionals and non professional, are both unaware of the work being done and the prevalence of the disease."[44] However, anything that could portray blacks as sickly or weak was also a potential threat. Thus, many Memphis blacks, who worried that the disease might be part of a conspiracy to further stain blacks as a race, did not accept Childs's efforts.

During his time in the clinic, Childs was also the target of some racial animus. Among his duties in the Gailor Clinic, he was a phlebotomist, who took blood samples from patients when directed to do so. Upon the complaint of a white female patient in the clinic, the Memphis fire and police commissioner, Joseph Boyle, referred to by some less flatteringly as "Holy" Joe Boyle, complained that a "nigger" was drawing blood from white patients. Crump's longstanding policy was not to interfere with the policies of the University of Tennessee, so Boyle's words ended up being more bluster than substance. Diggs characteristically did nothing, and nothing more came of the incident.[45]

Diggs needed technicians for work in the laboratories of the Sickle Cell Center and the blood bank, and apprenticing was something that he would undertake on his own. For example, in the late 1950s, he began training a Memphis rhythm-and-blues musician, Roosevelt Jamison, who graduated from the Stax Record Academy in 1956. Jamison became disillusioned with his musical career and began working as an orderly at the Gaston Hospital in October of that year. Diggs noticed his artistic ability and employed him to draw images of cells that Roosevelt observed through a microscope. It was probably through this relationship that Jamison became interested in becoming a laboratory technologist. There were no training programs for blacks and, as James Childs's experience with the white hospital patient showed, blacks in positions other than orderly could be controversial. Nevertheless, Jamison apprenticed with Diggs, who made Jamison a slide projectionist for his various lectures. By accompanying Diggs, Jamison would hear the lectures, and afterward Diggs would test him on their content. In this way, Jamison gained the training to become a laboratory technologist. In 1986, Diggs and Jamison met again at a book-signing party in Memphis for Peter Guralnick's rhythm-and-blues history: "Roosevelt hadn't seen him in a while, and he introduced me to Dr. Diggs excitedly ('You remember, I told you about Dr. Diggs!'), and despite an all-star turn out from the music world (Rufus Thomas, Solomon Burke, Sam Phillips, and David Porter, among others), Roosevelt spent most of his time with his one-time mentor and friend, reminiscing enthusiastically about old times."[46] Diggs was not a rhythm-and-blues aficionado per se, but he followed the people he worked with and knew with genuine interest.[47]

As the news of the center's efforts and reputation spread in the black community, more funds from local groups became available, which allowed Diggs's idea for a center to grow. Diggs was finally beginning to see a tangible outcome of his efforts at approximately the same time that Danny Thomas was campaigning to solicit funding for his hospital. Diggs worked together with D. B. Morrison in the Department of Laboratory Medicine. Part of the funding was used to send Diggs and his wife to Paris for an International Hematology Conference, at which he presented a paper on "The Sickle Cell Crisis."[48] By the late 1950s, Diggs was already managing a considerable number of sickle cell patients in the Memphis area who formed the basis of what would later become a sickle cell center. Patients were seen as sickle cell patients, but they could come to the clinic for any consultation or treatment. The center was only an outpatient clinic, and hence those requiring special or long-term care were referred either to another specialist or to the hospital.

The donation from the Herbert Herff Foundation was influential because it may have encouraged contributions by other citizens of Memphis, "mainly Blacks through social clubs, student and nursing organizations, church, labor and civic groups."[49] With the money provided by Herff and others, Diggs was able to hire another physician, Alfred Kraus, to work with him in the clinic. Fred, as he was known, was a trained hematologist from the University of Chicago. He was interested in the various medical activities at the University of Tennessee but had found a position at the Kennedy Hospital, located on Getwell Road.[50] He came to Memphis with his wife, Lorraine, who was a medical technologist. She used the opportunity to earn her doctorate at the university. It was unusual for a woman to pursue a doctorate, and so she had to be interviewed by the dean of the School of Graduate Health Sciences, Thomas Palmer Nash, before she could be admitted. Fred Kraus started working at the university in the mid-1950s. He was specifically interested in sickle cell as a clinical disease while his wife focused on the biomolecular aspects of the disease. Both Krauses were capable researchers in their own right.

By 1961 the support for sickle cell research had increased enough to create the core of the center that Diggs had in mind. In addition to Dr. Kraus, there was a fellow supported by a grant from St. Jude, a Japanese resident, and two technologists. The group was also publishing on sickle cell hemoglobin and remedies for the disease.[51] In the following year, the National Institutes of Health funded a one-year grant for fifty-seven thousand dollars, which was supplemented by local donations. The aim of the grant was to study chemical changes in sickle cell diseases at the time of vascular occlusion crisis, the primary complication of the disease.

In 1963 another doctor, Louis Barreras, was added to the center staff; he had fled his native Cuba to live in the United States. He had specialized in the blood diseases of children at the University of Havana, in particular in the management of acidosis. The Cuban Revolution produced many changes in the hospital where Barreras worked, but when he learned that the man who scrubbed the floors had been put in charge of the hospital, Barreras decided to leave. He told the authorities that his daughter had trouble with her spine, and that only a specialist in the United States could treat her. The Cuban authorities withheld Barreras's passport for four months until he promised to return after his daughter had received treatment. He agreed to this arrangement but had no intention of making good on his promise. As soon as his family was out of Cuba, he made his way to Ft. Lauderdale and from there to Memphis, where he could continue practicing medicine.[52]

The funds to hire Barreras, James Childs, the Krauses, and others came from increasingly diverse sources. The philanthropy of Herbert Herff and Danny Thomas helped, but money also came from big sources like the National Institutes of Health beginning in 1963 and continuing for ten years, the U.S. Public Health Service beginning in 1962 and continuing for four years, and from local groups. In 1962, the fifty-seven thousand dollars from the U.S. Public Health Service was used to hire Barreras, Iwao Iuchi from Japan as a hematology resident, Jeff Upshaw as a St. Jude Fellow, and Doris Sheldon as a technologist. In 1962 Ernestine Flowers and Maurice Tate joined the staff and would add to the knowledge about sickle cell in the home and at work; they would provide information that could be used to help patients adapt their illness to a more productive lifestyle by discovering the most effective way to treat the patient, the number of days lost in school or work, the risk of jobs and job training, and the best environment that would enable them to thrive. Part of the research conducted by the clinic included studying patients in their homes, which was at the heart of Diggs's goal, namely, "that the information will not only be beneficial to the physician treating the patient, but also to teachers, employers, health and welfare agencies, guidance councilors, and insurance companies."[53] In 1963, funding from the American Lebanese Syrian Associated Charities (ALSAC) was used for the creation of a Hematology Laboratory to study coagulation disorders, which was also supported by the University of Tennessee. The laboratory was staffed by another physician hired by Diggs, Marion Dugdale, a recent graduate of the Harvard Medical School.[54]

In addition to the prominent sources, there were also contributions from much smaller local groups of Negro churches, clubs, and business and professional leaders. Dr. Charles L. Dinkins, president of Owens College, donated twenty-one hundred dollars with the hope of increasing that amount in the future. Their efforts soon grew to thirty-seven hundred dollars.[55] Other black groups that participated in this effort included the Practical Nurses and the Cope Club. The Cope Club donated a carousel slide projector for education and outreach purposes. The money that these groups provided was raised at a variety of social events. The *Tri-State Defender,* Memphis's most prominent black newspaper, carried an appeal for more funds from the community. These efforts were made because the black community saw the value of what Diggs was doing and wanted to help maintain a continuity of service by the center at a time when funding was erratic. In 1966 similar local efforts led to the donation of two television sets for patients in the recently built William F. Bowld Hospital on the university campus.[56] Funds from local sources were also used to purchase wheelchairs. In 1968 the OsirUs Club hosted a fashion show to raise a hundred dollars for the center. This support by local black organizations represented progress in raising the awareness and understanding of sickle cell anemia, with the hope of finding a cure.

At the same time, some in the black community viewed Diggs's effort with suspicion. Some black leaders had concerns "that there was a certain stigma attached to sickle cell disease and that our [staff of the Sickle Cell Center] delving into it was a plot to make the race look bad."[57] The high rate of anemia among blacks was often cited as a reason to exclude them from the military and from working for the airlines. It was unwelcome news when the first black astronaut candidate was rejected from the space program to return to his regular U.S. Air Force duties.[58] The same thing happened during World War II when Diggs had to argue in favor of blacks possessing the trait to be allowed to perform regular but not stressful or high-altitude duties.[59]

In 1964 the American Society of Clinical Pathology honored Diggs with its Ward Burdick Award "in recognition of his meritorious contributions to the science of Clinical Pathology."[60] The medal was awarded in a ceremony at the society's annual meeting on October 1. Two years later the Volunteers in Aid of Sickle Cell Anemia, Inc., gave Diggs its Humanitarian Award "in recognition of his outstanding contributions and spirit of dedication in the field of sickle cell anemia."[61]

Just as Diggs found his work on the blood bank reflected in awards and the local media, he found the same thing happening with his work on sickle cell. Both local and national articles published in the late 1950s and 1960s reported Diggs's various efforts to support research and the work of the Sickle Cell Center, giving status and value to Diggs's efforts. He also began speaking more openly about the disease as it compared to other diseases. "Sickle cell disease," he is quoted in one newspaper article, "causes more paralysis and suffering than polio ever did."[62] He used any opportunity to provide information; such a statement also indicated his compassion for his patients and is a reminder of how much suffering he witnessed on virtually a daily basis. Diggs leveraged the growing interest to campaign for support on behalf of research.[63]

The work at the Sickle Cell Center focused on the structure of the hemoglobin molecule. Perhaps the center's most significant contribution was the discovery in 1966 of a new form of the sickle cell hemoglobin, which was quickly dubbed "Hemoglobin Memphis."[64] The discovery came when a sixty-year-old sickle cell patient caught the eye of Lorraine Kraus; this patient had a variation that seemed to make the disease less severe. Kraus wrote, "This hemoglobin variant in the alpha chain, when combined with sickle cell hemoglobin apparently makes sickle cell anemia a less severe disease."[65] What made this patient impressive were his age and the fact that he had the disease, but he experienced very few (if any) painful episodes. It was unusual for someone with the disease to live so long and to have such mild symptoms.[66]

Another significant contribution of the Sickle Cell Center was the investigation of carbamoyl phosphate, which altered the hemoglobin in patients so that the red cells did not sickle. However, despite the promise of the drug, it had undesirable side effects, such as neurological damage and cataracts found in test animals. Consequently, it had to be abandoned.[67]

The Sickle Cell Center in the 1960s and early 1970s was a growing organization. It was not always funded consistently, but it had enough money to hire the staff needed to do research and care for and study the patients in the program. The university provided the rooms for the center, and for this reason it was located in the Gailor Clinic. Although there was still little that could be done to ameliorate the effects of sickle cell, new ways were being found to detect it. Diggs participated in evaluating a new test produced by Orthro Diagnostics called Sickledex. It was simple enough for any laboratory technician to perform and read in five minutes, as compared to the standard sodium metabisulfate method, which was more complex and could take up to four hours to complete. Electrophoresis was still required to determine whether the cells under observation were from someone with the trait only or from someone with the anemia. Sickledex was also reported to have fewer false positives and false negatives, representing a real advantage for diagnosing and screening. Diggs participated in the promotion of the new invention by testing it in his laboratory and reporting the results.[68] He and his staff also tested Sickle-Sol by Dade, Sickle Quik by Schering, and Sickle-IS by Hyland—all found to be practical, readily available as screening procedures, and less expensive than hemoglobin electrophoresis tests. Diggs noted, "False positives and false negative tests could be reduced by the aggregation and separation modification with or without centrifugation."[69]

Diggs's Sickle Cell Center was able to follow the research and patient-care concerns that were most important to Diggs. He continued to see patients without charging for his services. The center studied children with various forms of sickle cell and thalassemia in the home, using normal children and children with the trait as a control. High-school football and basketball players with the trait were studied for two seasons in schools where the students were all African American. Some therapeutic progress was also made. While studying the ability of the kidney to tolerate acid load when ammonium chloride was given, painful crises were produced in nine of fourteen patients.[70] A plastic box was built, into which an ulcerated leg could be inserted, exposing it to an atmosphere of oxygen, which made it possible to obtain the healing of skin ulcers that did not respond to the usual forms of treatment. Papavirene was found to be beneficial in abdominal crises, but it had too many side effects to be practical.[71]

The home treatments of bone pain by warm fluids, hot baths, food, oral sodium citrate, and non-narcotic drugs were also useful, which helped to reduce the inconvenience and expense of emergency-room and hospital visits. Drugs that could lower respiration, such as opiates and their derivatives, were discouraged as dangerous because of the effect of lowered respiration on someone who was also anemic, because of the possibility of addiction, and because they were ineffective in reducing the worst pain during a crisis. Diuretics were also banned because dehydration could induce a crisis. As part of the educational mission of the center, a number of pamphlets and instructional programs were created under Diggs's supervision for parents, families, and patients. These materials were free to anyone and were distributed by the center for educational programs in schools and churches in Memphis and across the country.[72]

While Diggs was accustomed to dealing with racism in the clinic and laboratory, the civil rights movement outside was intruding on the work inside. Although a moderate, Diggs participated in the movement in Memphis in small ways. President Truman made civil rights a key doctrine of his administration, but there were already many grassroots efforts by African Americans for voting and equal education rights. Diggs wanted to include black doctors in mainstream medical professional organizations and to ensure that the disorders affecting blacks were not misappropriated to serve racist ends. Sickle cell anemia carried the stigma of racism, and Diggs had already learned to deal with it in the context of the university and the clinic. He wrote a letter to the editor of a Memphis newspaper in 1960, calling for the integration of the Memphis public libraries. Within the library system, blacks Memphians were allowed to visit only the Vance Avenue Negro Branch. They could request books from the main library and the other branches but were not allowed to visit them.[73] A year later he took another stand to end the discriminatory policy of the Memphis Zoo, which designated certain days when blacks could visit. The controversy over his acts led some to believe that he was under investigation by the FBI. His rejection of discrimination also led him to advocate for the hiring of Dr. Gene Stollerman, a Jew, to chair the Department of Medicine at a time when few Jewish physicians were on the faculty. Diggs threatened to resign from the university if Stollerman was not offered the position.[74] Whether his plea was influential remains unknown, but Stollerman was hired and had a highly successful career at the university.[75]

Diggs considered only a physician's credentials as necessary to practice. In 1956 he spoke before members of the Memphis and Shelby County Medical Society to argue that African American doctors should be included in the local professional groups affiliated with the American Medical Association. At this time the AMA did not prohibit black doctors from being members. However, it did require that, in order to be a member of the AMA, the applicant first had to be a member of a local AMA affiliate, which nearly always excluded black doctors. This latter condition prevented blacks from joining the AMA and led to the formation of a national black professional organization, the National Medical Association, which the AMA did not recognize.[76] Diggs felt compelled to try to convince his colleagues to remove the rule barring blacks locally.

His reasons were based on an appeal to the professional self-interest of his listeners and the need for better healthcare for all. "Colored doctors," he said, "cannot keep informed as well without the stimulus and guidance of their fellow physicians."[77] Black doctors could stay better informed about the latest medical advances and provide the best therapy to their patients only if they could network as white doctors did. As a debater, Diggs knew how to be persuasive; in a reference to the national healthcare insurance debate, he pointed out that including black doctors would help in "slowing down as much as possible governmental control."[78] More than this, however, Diggs wanted the local professional organization, the Memphis and Shelby County Medical Society, to be at the forefront of change: "The medical profession should take the lead in [honoring] professional skill and mental achievements."[79] Then, to emphasize the point, his last comment echoed an idea that would become familiar in civil rights rhetoric. "So that a man may be judged by what he knows and what he can do rather than by the color of his skin or where he lives."[80] He pointed out that the race line was already broken in sports and in the Army, and—just in case all of this might fail to convince his audience—he concluded his remarks with one last appeal: "Gentlemen—the Civil war is slightly over and we live in a world with Russia." At a time when America was experiencing a siege mentality based on the Cold War antagonism between the United States and the Soviet Union that pervaded national thinking, Diggs appealed to the need for national defense. The country should avail itself of all of its resources and make the most efficient use of them. There is no record of the response to his comments, but it is unlikely that many opinions were swayed.

At the same time that Diggs was debating with members of his own profession, he felt the need to respond to a question about racial separation, which used sickle cell anemia as a key instrument for segregation. Here he was on familiar grounds, but the issue came from a nonprofessional direction. In September of 1957, Diggs responded to a letter from Robert B. Patterson, who was at this time executive secretary of the Association of Citizens' Councils in Greenwood, Mississippi. With its call for "racial integrity and states rights," this white association and others like it grew out of the backlash among some southern whites to the Supreme Court's *Brown v. Board of Education of Topeka* decision of 1954 and very likely was loosely affiliated with the Ku Klux Klan.[81] Patterson's letter to Diggs is lost, so it can only inferred from Diggs's response that Patterson was seeking Diggs's support for a statement that the sickle cell anemia is "an indication of racial inferiority of the negro race,"[82] or, as Diggs interpreted it, that sickle cell anemia was a reason "for or against integration or segregation."[83]

Diggs described himself as "a physician who is concerned with the health of all people, regardless of race or color and as a loyal Southerner, who does not consider it an honor to be asked to participate in propaganda of this type."[84] He expressed his disgust at being queried in this way, and underscored that study into understanding sickle cell anemia "would be gravely interfered with if the Citizens' Councils placed emphasis on sickle cell disease in their published information or whispering campaigns."[85] Diggs pointed out to Patterson that people with any hereditary disease should not intermarry, and that some form of sickle cell disease, such as thalassemia affecting Mediterranean people or hereditary spherocytosis affecting Teutonic people, can be found in different races. "One might therefore, with equal accuracy, argue that intermarriage would degrade the Negro race."[86] The use of the *reductio ad absurdum* argument is an example of Diggs's debating skill that he further punctuates with a rhetorical flourish in the closing paragraph, "I would not recommend that the Citizens' Councils play the 'sickle cell string,' for the notes will be discordant and will be as distasteful to the ears of reasonable and fair-minded white people as it will be unfair and hurtful to colored people."[87] In his blunt but even-handed way, Diggs does not argue against racism by advocating for a more diverse and inclusive world than Patterson seems to imagine, but for a world that in Diggs's view simply would not include racism as an object in it. Though his words were measured, he made his point: "It's a medical problem, not a racial problem." Years later, when he recalled his feeling toward the letter, he said more bluntly: "I told them to go to hell."[88]

As the issues of racism in medicine and public life became more strident and unavoidable in the middle and late 1960s, Diggs's sense of southern moderation began to change. He could no longer remain silent about the major issues of the day. The request for support from the Association of Citizens' Councils and the concern about the "image" of sickle cell research were forcing him to become more partisan, as evidenced by his presentation to the Memphis Medical Society.

Like everyone else, Diggs was stunned by the assassination of Dr. Martin Luther King Jr. on April 4, 1968. In an unpublished letter to the editors, he wrote a response to a *Time* editorial: "The majority of citizens of Memphis deeply regret the ruthless slaying of Martin Luther King."[89] He was taken aback by the characterization of the city as a "Southern backwater," a "decaying Mississippi river town,"[90] and of its mayor as "intransigent."[91] Diggs was distressed by the assertion that the mayor had caused the situation by a failure "to meet the modest wage and compensation demand," which was the immediate reason for the return of Dr. King, "the conqueror of Montgomery, Birmingham and Selma."[92] His response to what happened in Memphis in early April and late May of that year was deeply personal. The unions struck the City Hospital, which left only doctors and nurses to care for the patients; all licensed practical nurses, orderlies, and staff members refused to work, which meant that all of the duties of the hospital—from kitchen to laundry to ward cleanups—had to be performed by the doctors, residents, and nurses. By the time he wrote this letter, the unions had been on strike at the John Gaston Hospital for fifty-nine days. Some patients were still admitted, but the emergency room was closed, which may have contributed to the short duration of the strike because new patients that were undesirable to the private hospitals had to be diverted to the other Memphis hospitals. Residents maintained a good attitude for a time, but they began to complain that the length of the strike was undermining their education, so places were found for them in other hospitals. Some of the

Gaston patients were moved to the nearby Veterans Affairs Hospital while the remainder were transferred to the other private hospitals in town.[93]

As terrible as Dr. King's assassination was, the editorial failed, in Diggs's view, to make anything but a passing reference to the ensuing breakdown in civil, legal, and governmental order that was also part of the story. This troubled Diggs so much that he sought to restore that balance in his letter to *Time*. The editorial presented the events in Memphis from the point of view of the assassination and ensuing violence, but, Diggs points out, it said nothing about the union that "ordered an illegal strike of the Sanitation Workers against the City of Memphis, dictated the amount of salary raise required and insisted on a dues check-off."[94] As Diggs saw it, the editorial described the labor dispute leading up to King's death as a minor one until, in Diggs's words, "it became hidden by the smoke and fire of racial violence."[95] The editorial told only half of the story, namely the events leading up to and immediately following King's death, but said nothing of the illegality of the strike or the lack of consideration that the "funds of a municipality belong to the people and not to the Mayor."[96] As Diggs wrote, "There is good reason for municipal employees to organize and to develop a machinery (union) for presenting their grievances and needs. They also have a right to resign as individuals or as a group. The city or other governmental agency on the other hand must reserve the right and the obligation to maintain services for the good of the community as a whole and to fill positions vacated as soon as possible."[97]

That Diggs was deeply troubled by the events surrounding April 4 is clear. He, the hospital and medical community, and the city were shaken to their foundations by what had happened, and everyone had to find a way to make sense of it. Diggs's sense of moderation instinctively sought to find the middle ground between the right of the workers to form a union and make their grievances known to their employer and the city government's need to not give in to extra-governmental pressure.

Diggs's political and social attitude as a moderate changed in the aftermath of King's assassination, the extended hospital strike, and the ensuing riots around the country. He was no longer comfortable with waiting for cooler heads to prevail. He could be patient with the policy requiring the segregation of blood units, and even with the time it took for the growth of the Sickle Cell Center. He was well aware of the problem of racism, but he also believed the problem was so complex that it could only be resolved gradually. By the late 1960s, however, the political and social pressures were such that gradual improvement was no longer an option, and he began to take a more active role in the improvement of his country.

By December 1969, Diggs was ready to retire from the university, though not from any of the duties that preoccupied him. He was as interested as ever in solving the mysteries of sickle cell anemia and seeing the Sickle Cell Center grow; the workload for his retirement would be very much the same as before. The center was staffed and functioning, with Alfred Kraus as an excellent researcher who was able to take over the director's duties.

In a 1968 newspaper article, Diggs observed: "We have about 1000 sickle cell victims from the Memphis area in our files and are following about 300 of them very closely. They come to us for free treatment when they are not in trouble [too ill to come to the center]."[98] Diggs's sickle cell patients could come to the clinic for any reason, and this meant that the clinic's staff would be able to see them under a variety of circumstances. The advances made in understanding the disease were generally meager, but Diggs noted that the center was able to stay ahead of the research literature most of the time. He also noted with candor that, "compared to the problem, that's not saying much."[99] His biggest disappointment was that little had changed regarding treatment: "We are able to spare them [the patients] a lot of pain, save a few lives temporarily and spot some cases early enough to head off some complications. We have found that big doses of a vasodilator (a drug that improves circulation by expanding blood vessels) and avoiding dehydration and acidosis is the best treatment."[100] Diggs noted that in 1910 the average life expectancy of sickle cell sufferers was fourteen years of age, and that by 1968 the life expectancy had not changed. Just as he did with the blood bank in 1945, he was ready to watch the Sickle Cell Center take its first steps into the world while he stepped back to play a more supportive role that would allow more time for research. The advantage for him would be to continue exploring the natural history of the disease with fewer of the daily concerns of running the center. What he could not anticipate was the degree to which these problems would increase as he and the center entered the 1970s.

I have loved no darkness, sophisticated no truth,
nursed no delusion, allowed not fear.
—Sir William Osler quoting Matthew Arnold

Chapter 6
Retirement

The beginning of 1971 seemed to promise the recognition and long-sought financial support for the Diggs Sickle Cell Center. In February, President Richard M. Nixon in his "Special Message to the Congress Proposing a National Health Strategy" surprised everyone when he declared sickle cell anemia to be a target for research, affirming that $6,000,000 would be designated in the following fiscal year for research to end the disease.[1] At the time, it seemed an unexpected gesture of federal largesse, but it was based on a sea change in American politics away from the programs of President Lyndon Johnson's "Great Society" legislation and toward a more fiscally and politically conservative Republicanism. President Nixon rode this political wave into office with the promise to curtail what he characterized as the runaway spending of Democrats. In supporting sickle cell research, he was motivated by principle as well as by pragmatic considerations. His speech addressed the growing concern that national healthcare costs were spiraling out of control. One way to bring costs down, he argued, was by promoting health maintenance organizations (HMOs) in urban and remote rural areas, which would focus on health promotion rather than disease prevention, and by reducing the number of malpractice claims and lowering the cost of malpractice insurance. Cancer research received an increase in funding. However, to everyone's surprise, sickle cell was singled out as a new research area that deserved federal support, addressing the criticism that the government was indifferent to the healthcare problems of black Americans and, at the same time, deflecting attention away from his proposal to significantly reduce the overall budget for the National Institutes of Health after "excessive spending" during Johnson's presidency.

Nixon's proposal did not provide new money for sickle cell research, but rather took the funding from reductions in other research programs. One newspaper reporter noted that "only now is sickle-cell anemia beginning to get even a fraction of the attention it deserves and black power at last is the reason why."[2] Cardiovascular researchers saw their funding decline and resented the intrusion of politics into research matters.[3] Others pointed out the incongruity of the choice of research on sickle cell over, for example, hypertension. It was also pointed out that sickle cell research was related to other hematology studies already underway, and could be incorporated into those existing programs without the need for creating a new research category. "Ironically, hypertension is a far worse killer of blacks than sickle-cell anemia, so in the long run Mr. Nixon has done black America no great favor with this little instance of robbing Peter to pay Paul for Dick's benefit."[4] Nevertheless, in August of that year, Congress passed an amendment to the Public Health Service Act that established sickle cell as an inherited disease. The secretary of the Department of Health, Education, and Welfare created the National Sickle Cell Disease Advisory Board in August, which would set up a program to make grants and contracts available for the development of voluntary screening and counseling programs primarily through other existing programs, such as the one already operating in Memphis.[5]

The president's announcement transformed sickle cell research almost overnight into a national issue and for the first time made it widely known to the nation. In 1972 the disease was featured in the film *A Warm December* directed by and starring Sidney Poitier; sickle cell was also featured on two popular television shows, *M*A*S*H* and *Marcus Welby, M.D.* Two hundred sports figures, including Willie Stargel and Dock Ellis of the Pittsburgh

Pirates baseball team and boxer Muhammad Ali, lent their names to attracting attention and money to the cause of ending the disease by having all blacks screened for the genetic abnormality.[6] If there was no cure, then perhaps genetic counseling could provide a solution.

Before all of these events came into play, Diggs had been building and organizing the Sickle Cell Center with a patchwork of support from 1958 to 1971 with the contribution of a few rooms from the university and financial support from the American Lebanese and Syrian Associated Charities (ALSAC, the fundraising arm of the St. Jude Children's Research Hospital), Herbert Herff, a National Institutes of Health grant, and other local groups that contributed through fundraising events. This was enough for him to modestly equip and staff what would become the research facility. Funding from the National Institutes of Health provided continuous support for and expansion of the center from 1962 until 1973. As with the blood bank in the late 1930s, Diggs had a free hand to design and operate the center according to his best judgment, which meant that it both provided laboratory support for the care of sickle cell patients and worked to learn from the illnesses of those admitted to the hospital.

With the infusion of new funding to support the Sickle Cell Center came federal regulations. Diggs and his colleagues quickly began to feel the unintended consequences of the federal bill and the complex pressures of civil rights in the 1970s. The new bill, called the Comprehensive Sickle Cell Center Grant, changed the structure of the center as Diggs conceived it by requiring that 60 percent of the funding be used for community services, including employing nonprofessional staff members, and the remaining 40 percent to be used for employing health professionals and conducting research. Education and research went hand-in-hand, often overlapping at the center, but the focus had always been on educating the patient and not on outreach to the community. This new grant separated the two functions without any clear guidelines as to how this would be done, and made education an outreach function. In addition, the new funding required the employment of additional staff for which there were no job descriptions, no apparent need in Diggs's view, and no provision for training. This uncertainty was compounded by the loss of the previous NIH grant supporting the Sickle Cell Center, with the result that one professional's job had to be terminated. Diggs assumed incorrectly that the previous grant, which had supported the medical-care portion of the center up to that point, would continue alongside the new one. In effect, he and the center's staff would have to recalibrate themselves and their services to fit these new guidelines.[7]

The federal bill also provided benefits for the center, such as training of new nonprofessionals in administrative matters, increasing public awareness on the frequency and symptoms of sickle cell, and training staff to help with education, counseling, and screening projects. But the program design stipulated by the grant did not fit Diggs's idea of how the scientific organization should be structured. It created a working environment that did not operate smoothly and was a source of dissatisfaction to everyone involved for the first few years under the new guidelines.

Changes to the center required by the new federal grant led to the creation in 1971 of a Memphis Regional Sickle Cell Council (MRSCC), composed mainly of the parents of sickle cell patients and other laypeople. It was created to assist in the application of the money that would fund a comprehensive sickle cell center in Memphis. The purposes of this new council were to aid in finding new grant support for research, to support local fundraising efforts, and to inform the public about the disease.[8] Another group, the Memphis Research Coordinating Committee, was organized to enhance communications between the Memphis Regional Sickle Cell Council and the research community in Memphis and elsewhere, but by 1974 the council was struggling to develop as an organization. It was not meeting with the other agencies with which it was supposed to coordinate efforts, its representatives failed to attend scheduled meetings, and there were no provisions for the election of a new liaison committee.[9]

Diggs became frustrated with the overlapping responsibilities, the seemingly artificial dichotomies, the confrontations and accusations, the personality clashes, the poor communication, and the unwillingness to compromise—all of which resulted in an uncomfortable work environment. There was even a rumor that someone in the Sickle Cell Center was reporting on activities in the center to a local minister who was critical of its work.[10] Grant requirements that blacks could work only in areas that were separated from those of the professional staff caused much of the tension. This separation of the research and educational components of the center and the requirement for the newly hired employees to conform to university regulations were contrary to Diggs's idea of an optimally run organization: "The required separation of the program into a community arm and an institutional (University) arm and the creation of new positions to be filled entirely by Blacks favored polarization along racial lines."[11] The situation led to a "town and gown" or a "people vs. the establishment" situation that was also a reflection of the larger civil rights unrest of the 1960s and 1970s.

The successes of the movement during the Johnson presidency included the Civil Rights Act of 1964, which prohibited discrimination by race, ethnicity, minority status, and gender; followed by the Voting Rights Act of 1965, which prohibited discrimination in voting; and Medicare, which provided health insurance for those over sixty-five years of age but also spurred racial integration of hospitals by making payments conditional on desegregation. The legislative changes of this period represented significant changes. On the ground, however, the changes were not so apparent. In 1968 Martin Luther King was assassinated in Memphis, and in 1972 the ugly revelation of the Tuskegee Syphilis Study that had been supported by the U.S. Public Health Service for forty years added to the feeling that the racial structures of Jim Crow still seemed to be in place despite the legislative successes. Stokely Carmichael started the call for "Black Power" both as a way to unite blacks and as a critique of nonviolence as proposed by Martin Luther King. The civil rights movement was evolving and becoming more demanding in its desire for real change in the way African Americans were treated at all levels of government and in all facets of everyday life. There was growing suspicion among blacks over what the "true" intentions of sickle cell screening might be.[12] Diggs resented the intrusion into what he saw as the essential mission of the center: "Individuals who are engaged in research should not be penalized by being forced to assume the impossible and Herculean task of having to solve racial, social, economic and other community problems in order to obtain funds for their investigations."[13]

As he had learned and practiced ever since his student days at Hopkins and Rochester, Diggs knew all too well that the limited time given to researchers should be spent "in the laboratory and in the library rather than around council tables discussing administrative and community matters."[14] He was unhappy that the center had moved away from its research and patient care mission. He exclaimed: "Community problems need to be solved but the burden of their solution should not be saddled on members of the faculty of one section of one department of one college of the University of Tennessee Center for the Healthy Sciences."[15]

If there were problems, there were also glimmers of light for Diggs and the center. The school busing program in Memphis—part of the process to desegregate school systems resulting from the *Brown v. Board of Education* Supreme Court decision of 1954—offered an opportunity to educate the public about the nature of sickle cell. Diggs knew it was not enough to simply inform the general public. Key people, such as white teachers, who might not have experience with children with sickle cell, needed to be instructed. In 1972, the Memphis Regional Sickle Cell Council worked with Parent Teacher Associations and high-school principals to inform them not only of what the disease was, but to make them aware of the ways in which it might manifest itself. The goal was to ensure that students with the disease were recognized and helped, not ignored or mistreated. Sometimes a teacher might categorize a student as lazy when in fact he or she was not feeling well on the day in question. Likewise, coaches should understand that the strenuous exercises they assigned their athletes could lead to low oxygen, which in a child with sickle cell might cause a crisis.[16] The outcome of this effort is unclear, but it allowed Diggs and the staff to challenge many misconceptions about the disease and its genetic origins. This was the kind of outreach that Diggs considered part of the center's mission, and yet, under the guidelines of the new grant, it represented a time-consuming distraction.

Instead of focusing on the sick, the staff of the Sickle Cell Center saw their energy divided between research and education as separate activities, something that ran counter to Diggs's viewpoint: "The medical care of patients and the conduct of laboratory procedures and the research activities of necessity have to be located where facilities, equipment and specialty services are available. The Community portion of the program ideally should also be located in the same building so that communication can be facilitated and full use made of educational resources."[17] The MRSCC was located on Southern Avenue, about three miles from the medical center. "We could not have planned, if we tried, a system that was more destined to cause trouble and to fail than the dichotomous (double headed Monster) system that was established. One cannot expect to win a football game with two quarterbacks calling plays at the same time. 'A wheel cannot turn on two axles.'"[18] When Diggs reflected on the agitation caused by government regulations and social issues, his displeasure was palpable.

Despite the challenges, Diggs continued his investigation into sickle cell's underlying mechanism, and the center continued its search for ways to ameliorate the disease. With his emeritus status, Diggs was much less involved with the center's day-to-day operations and so was able to spend more time on research and patient care. Along with Ernestine Flowers, he continued to investigate the natural history of the disease and activities related to it in the home. During this period they were working with forty-five families affected by the disease.[19] Their work explored the multifaceted nature of sickle cell anemia, involving how it could affect each individual patient differently in personal, financial, and social ways. Diggs believed that those with sickle cell were handicapped, but that they should also be able to support themselves rather than be dependent on others. But he recommended that people with sickle cell should be employed in jobs that avoided situations that could cause a crisis.[20]

Harvey Itano and Linus Pauling identified sickle cell as a genetic abnormality with an identifiable location in the body, namely, the globin portion of hemoglobin. Without an intervention that would cure or at least control the disease, many people thought that the best way to eliminate sickle cell was to prevent the genetic defect from being transmitted from parent to child. With the announcement by President Nixon of sickle cell as a target of national concern, many healthcare professionals and politicians considered requiring that all blacks be tested for the disease, and that they either be counseled against marriage, or that marriage licenses be refused to those testing positive for sickle cell. Genetics seemed to offer a way to eliminate the disease; at first, many people supported this view, including black organizations, such as the Black Panthers.[21] By the mid-1970s, Tennessee and other states had enacted or were considering laws embodying this attitude.

Considerable confusion existed over the difference between sickle cell anemia and the sickle cell trait. Some of these laws were predicated on the assumption that both anemia and the trait were a single disease,[22] a serious misunderstanding that Diggs had tried to clarify for forty years. He recognized in his earliest writing that there was a clear distinction between the trait and the disease, and that the trait was compatible with normal life. He saw screening as a means to inform and council patients, but not as a means to control a group of people. Many, but most notably Pauling himself, advocated mass screenings of anyone of African descent in order to identify carriers and to restrict or prevent their marriage or procreation. Pauling famously advocated marking sickle cell carriers with a tattoo on the forehead to identify them. In this way, carriers of the defective gene would easily recognize each other and be discouraged from marrying, or encouraged to have fewer children or, with a simple blood test to determine the presence of the gene in a fetus, opt for an abortion.[23] The outcry that ensued was widespread. Accusations of genocide and eugenics were levied, and reports were published of people with sickle cell being fired from their jobs, or being denied employment or insurance, and of students with the trait being told not to participate in sports. Thus the disease continued to carry a stigma of sickliness and racial inferiority. Some people began to wonder if mass screening singled out those who tested positive for ostracism at school or work, based on the widespread confusion over the difference between the disease and the trait. Critics wondered whether screening would serve the purposes of genetics or genocide. The backlash to the screening laws led to the repeal of many of those laws.[24]

Diggs was aware of the social controversy and the backlash from the black community, and of the views of Pauling and others. He rejected universal screening of blacks from the beginning on ethical grounds. He noted this in a letter to the editor of the *New England Journal of Medicine*: "Genetic counseling to prevent the carrier form of the disease, the sickle-cell trait without anemia (Hb A-S), is not reasonable, but advice and guidance in family planning is indicated when both parents have abnormalities that may be transmitted to produce a chronic, serious and disabling disease."[25] Any major effort to eliminate the disease, he believed, should be put into education, research, and medical care, not into "marking" an entire race: "The future hope of any hereditary disease is in genetic counseling, but this requires the training of genetic counselors who are well versed in the laws of biology and heredity and who are experts in human relations."[26]

The field of genetic counseling was changing in the early 1970s as it moved away from a prescriptive, eugenics-oriented practice based on clinical science to a more client-centered stance that focused on the patient's options.[27] Diggs believed that genetic counseling should be voluntary for both marital partners, and they should be allowed to use the information in any way they chose: "One should never tell an individual what to do. The individual should be given the facts and leave it up to the person to choose what he or she wished to do. Genetic counseling and family planning are often misinterpreted as racial genocide, which of course is ridiculous, for it is the disease and not the counseling that is genocide."[28] Avoiding the birth of children with the severest form of the disease, sickle cell anemia, he noted elsewhere, was "genosave."[29] He knew of the controversy, and of the resistance that most people felt about being counseled. But this situation, he believed, would change: "In the future, counseling will have top priority, but at present it should be played with a soft key."[30]

Since sickle cell was very likely linked as an adaptive prophylactic against malaria, the key property of the disease should not be the color of a person's skin, but the region of the world where malaria is prevalent. As Diggs expressed it, "There is no more reason for considering that prevention of births of babies with sickle-cell anemia among Negroes is black genocide than that prevention of propagation of children by carriers of thalassemia, hemophilia, Tay-Sachs or Pelger-Huët disease, or other hereditary disease that occur predominantly among whites is white genocide."[31] After all, he would argue, "the statistical chance that both parents will have the trait is approximately 1 per cent, rather than 8 to 10 percent."[32] Nevertheless, the consequences of producing a child with sickle cell anemia were devastating for the child and the parents, and Diggs saw the appropriate role that counseling would play in advising the parents of their options, not to tell them what option to choose. When he saw screening move away from a position of universal application, he chose to let it run its course until more reasonable heads could prevail.

Given the changes that genetic counseling was undergoing, it is not difficult to see how the added attention to sickle cell research increased confusion over the disease and its sufferers. Diggs pointed out that testers often did not sufficiently inform those who were tested as to what it was they were being tested for and, when the results were positive, they were not properly informed of what the results meant. Forty years earlier, he had argued that the trait was consistent with a normal life, but often it was still confused with the anemia, which led to "unjustified anxiety and fears, increased insurance rates and coverage, unemployment, and denial [of] educational and recreational opportunities."[33] Compulsory testing was required by law by many states before issuing marriage licenses. According to Diggs, this practice was misguided, because the black population could not be defined by physical features, and because sickle cell also occurred in those of Turkish, Spanish, Greek, Italian, Arabian, and Indian ancestry.

"In summary," he wrote in 1978 to a Mississippi nursing student, "it is my opinion that mass screening and financing of mass screening by tax funds is no longer justified and should be banned."[34] Diggs was not opposed to testing or to screening for individuals requesting the information, but did feel strongly that testing should be done on a voluntary basis and only to help individuals, not to attempt to cure a race.

Despite the controversy, Diggs had reason for satisfaction in the growth of St. Jude. He stayed in touch with Danny Thomas, who continued to express his appreciation for Diggs's role in the creation of the hospital. Thomas wrote: "I am particularly grateful that you wrote about our interest in sickle cell anemia, and how far back you go with it, because I was having some trouble trying to convince a few of the black personalities in show business that through you we were in truth pioneers in the fight against that disease which seems to strike their race especially."[35] In 1975 the St. Jude Board of Directors appointed Diggs to their National Advisory Board.[36]

Throughout his career, Diggs sought to maintain a comprehensive understanding of whatever interested him by accumulating and reading everything that was published about it. This was especially true of sickle cell anemia and blood banking. In his own publications, he typically included a summary of what was known about a topic he proposed to address, a feature of his writing that was also reflected in his thorough reference lists. By 1981 he completed the task that he had started in 1929 of compiling every article in any language that he could find on sickle cell disease. It took nearly a year to assemble and organize the over three thousand articles, reprints, and, in some cases, typescript copies of articles from 1910 to 1970. The year 1970 was likely chosen because of the dramatic public profile of the disease beginning in 1971. The volumes were bound with the help of the Bluff City Medical Society Auxiliaries, which was made up of the wives of the black doctors in Memphis that constituted its membership. The Auxiliaries raised fifteen hundred dollars to bind the paper articles and to have the set reproduced on microfilm and microfiche. A bound collection of sixty-four volumes was presented to the University of Tennessee Mooney Library. Additional sets were made for the Armed Forces Institute of Pathology and for the National Library of Medicine.[37] The articles were also reproduced on microfilm and microfiche and given to Morehouse College, Howard University Medical School, and Meharry University Medical School.[38]

On April 11, 1972, the Southern Christian Leadership Conference honored Diggs at a dinner in Philadelphia by giving him its Martin Luther King Medical Achievement Award. Humanitarian awards were also included in the presentations. The event was a hundred-dollar-per-plate affair at which twenty-eight other recipients were also recognized. Coretta Scott King made the presentation of the awards. In 1978 the Virginia Press Association honored Diggs with its Virginian of the Year Award.[39] He enjoyed the acknowledgment from his home state, and also the opportunity to return to the places where he had grown up and to visit with old friends.

In 1985 Diggs was startled to read in the local paper that the St. Jude organization was reevaluating Memphis as a location for its hospital in favor of moving to the Washington Medical School in St. Louis. He was doubly surprised because he read it first in the newspaper, and because he was unaware that St. Jude was even considering such a move. The loss of St. Jude to the city was apparent to him, but more than that it would represent the loss of a second vital venue for conducting research into a cure for sickle cell anemia. By 1982 he was no longer on the St. Jude National Advisory Board, and after 1975 he was no longer on the St. Jude Board of Directors. Although no longer engaged in the political discussions related to St. Jude, the dramatic announcement on the front page of the *Commercial Appeal* immediately summoned his instinct to protect St. Jude. In part, this was born of the tension that existed between St. Jude and the university in the 1960s, in which Diggs was personally involved: the vexing issue was whether St. Jude should be an independent research institution or should be "tied" to a university, and whether the hospital would thrive in another city.

Diggs was no doubt expressing some of the frustration experienced at the Sickle Cell Center after it was reorganized in 1972. He wrote a short letter to the editors of the *Commercial Appeal*:

> The individual members of the St. Jude scientific investigative staff and the professional departments of the St. Jude Children's Research Hospital should remain free to follow their own research leads. They should be allowed to plan to conduct their activities in a manner that, to them, seems best. They should not be dominated by Washington University, the University of Tennessee or by any other institution. They should not be forced to follow protocols established by committees other than their own. For the sake of the future health, happiness and prolongation of live of children with diseases not considered to be

catastrophic, St. Jude should remain as an independent and autonomous unit. Research of all types basic, bio-medical and applied, should not be submerged or lost in any university complex, regardless of how big, prestigious and rich the absorbing institution may be.[40]

Diggs believed without question that St. Jude should remain in Memphis as an independent and autonomous unit. He believed in its research-driven and donor-funded model, its strong patient-care orientation, and its position as the second location in the city for sickle cell research. He felt this so strongly that he believed it would be better for St. Jude to leave Memphis than to stay and compromise its core values. St. Jude, he felt, should continuously evaluate its position and, if circumstances warranted, move to whichever location would provide fertile soil for it to thrive. The essence of St. Jude, he would write to another St. Jude advocate, was in the substantial support it received as a research hospital and the quality of care its patients received. Diggs's belief in St. Jude remained as steadfast as ever, and he was relieved in February of 1986 when the St. Jude Board of Directors agreed that the hospital would remain in Memphis.[41]

After his retirement, Diggs continued his daily schedule in the office. Although no longer administratively involved in the operation of the center, he was involved in the salient issues being considered there, in performing research, and in seeing patients. In late 1987 he was diagnosed with an intestinal malignancy, which was surgically removed. The tumor did not appear to migrate to any other part of his body. After the operation he informed his colleagues that he would be working at home and to contact him there, but he also reassured them that he was staying active by riding tractors, sawing wood, picking up pecans, and writing about sickle cell. Beatrice continued to help with his library work and typing.[42]

In 1985 the university created several endowments, including one it called the Lemuel Whitley Diggs Professorship in Medicine. Diggs's reputation grew with each award and honor. He started receiving mail from individuals asking for advice. Schoolchildren asked him for information about sickle cell anemia that they could use in their assignments.[43] Occasionally he would hear from parents asking him to review a child's clinical records and comment on the quality of care the child was receiving.[44] In each case he replied with his usual care and completeness, for he viewed each correspondence as an educational opportunity to talk about sickle cell. He also corresponded with colleagues about events and people in their past. In recognition of his many awards, Diggs also received notes from congressmen from Tennessee, Virginia, and New York. One message came from Hugh Scott of Pennsylvania, who knew Diggs from his student days at Randolph-Macon College: "Can it be 66 years since you got me off the hook, after I'd invited two different girls to Commencement? The one I took, I kept—and still have after all this time."[45]

In another letter, he summarized what he had learned in over fifty years of experience as the best treatment of the leg ulcers that are a common complication of sickle cell. He started by reflecting on the range of remedies that had been tried over the years: "These have included antiseptic and antibiotic solutions, powders, salves and ointments of various types, vasodilator drugs, anticoagulants, proteolytic enzymes, table sugar, dressings consisting of clots of the patients own blood, cod liver oil, elastic sponges, bed rest, transfusions, oxygen chamber and pinch and full thickness skin grafts."[46] Patients without access to healthcare and often in desperation tried to treat themselves with "carbolated Vaseline, axle grease, crank case oil, shoe polish, turpentine and kerosene."[47] In the end, however, he found that the most effective treatments were the simplest and the least expensive. "The best treatment in my opinion is soap, water and sterile dressings and the avoidance of strong medications of any kind."[48] Cost was important, Diggs was saying, but even more critical was the need to educate people to care for themselves rather than depend on care given in a doctor's office or the hospital.

In 1991 Diggs received the Outstanding Citizen Award from the Civitan Clubs, a volunteer service organization.[49] He received many congratulatory notes from colleagues, administrators, and friends, including one recorded by Danny Thomas acknowledging Diggs's role in the formation and early direction of St. Jude Children's Research Hospital: "Through the years and even in retirement, if you can call his busy schedule that, Dr. Diggs has been a truly invaluable mentor, counselor, and friend of St. Jude."[50] The recognition came with a proclamation from the mayor, declaring April 4, 1991, as Lemuel W. Diggs Day in the city of Memphis.

One of the most poignant moments for Diggs in these later years was the retirement in 1991 of one of his closest colleagues at the University of Tennessee, Ann Bell. For both Lemuel and Beatrice, it was emotional.

"One of the best of many good things," he wrote Bell, "was your employment as 'Secretary' in the Department of Clinical Pathology, as it was then called, soon after your graduation with a BS degree from Randolph Macon College for women (1941)."[51] He then recalled the steps of her career at the university, including the students, the workshops, and the publications, especially *The Morphology of Human Blood Cells*, then in its fifth edition.[52] Beatrice wrote a letter that included a recollection of their trips together and the work that Ann had done with Dorothy Sturm to create the watercolor images for the department and for the book. Ann responded to Beatrice first, thanking her and crediting her and Diggs with supporting her throughout her career.[53] Five days later she wrote to Diggs, describing the steps in her career and attributing each of them to his mentoring and support. Upon being asked to coauthor the *Morphology*, she had said: "What a triumvirate we made as we produced five editions for Abbott!"[54] Bell expressed difficulty in finding the words to express her feelings. "You [Beatrice] and Dr. Diggs made me feel that I belonged to the Diggs family and that has made me very happy for all of these years that we have worked together."[55] Ann would continue to work part-time at the university, but she devoted the remainder of her life to organizing and preserving Diggs's intellectual legacy.

Diggs remained active in his communications with colleagues and friends. In 1993 he entered the fray of the national healthcare reform debate led by Hillary Rodham Clinton. He sent three broad recommendations to the Task Force on National Health Care Reform. The first was to teach interns and residents the costs of the diagnostic, prognostic, and therapeutic procedures that they ordered for their patients, and to educate the public that, because cost is a factor, patients cannot automatically expect every procedure to be performed that might diagnostically be beneficial. Diggs's second recommendation was that rationing of healthcare services, as unpalatable as it seemed, would be necessary where resources were scarce or extremely expensive. In the third he emphasized that taxpayers should be responsible for essential and relatively inexpensive procedures, but not nonessential or elective procedures.[56] Diggs sent copies of his recommendations to colleagues; they were received warmly, and he also received a brief acknowledgment from the White House.[57] As he had done fifty years earlier in 1943, Diggs argued in favor of medical reform on the grounds that it should in some ways change to conform with the larger social circumstances in which medicine had to operate. But he also continued to believe in the need for individual responsibility for at least part of the cost of this care, and some rationing of expensive and scarce resources. The doctor-patient relationship and the principle of treating each patient as a unique individual remained at the heart of his professional beliefs. At the same time, he preferred to see healthcare costs managed locally.

In late December of 1994, Diggs's health began to decline. He remained as active as possible, even planning and writing another article on sickle cell. He was thinking about the importance of postmortem examinations to "establish the cause of death and to discover new anatomical facts."[58] Diggs was active until about three weeks before his birthday, when he began to have trouble swallowing. He remained in bed and appeared to be near his end. However, in defiance of the inevitable, he lingered until his birthday on January 9, when he stopped breathing. "I think he really wanted to live to be 95," his daughter Alice observed.[59]

On the following day, the newspapers carried extensive stories about Diggs's life and achievements, each with a slightly different view. The *Commercial Appeal* mentioned sickle cell but focused on the blood bank, St. Jude, his many awards, and comments by his friends and colleagues.[60] An editorial in the same issue reflected this perspective. By contrast, the *Tri-State Defender* mentioned Diggs's awards but focused primarily on his lifelong effort to understand and treat sickle cell anemia, his commitment to the physical, psychological, and social well-being of his patients, and his willingness to challenge segregation laws by training black technicians.[61]

The funeral service for Lemuel Whitley Diggs was held on January 14, 1995, at the Church of the River, the First Unitarian Church of Memphis. Those who spoke at the service were Howard Horn, who had been named L. W. Diggs Alumni Professor of Medicine at the University of Tennessee; Ann Bell; Andrewnetta Hawkins Jones, a former employee; Dan Brookoff, a hematologist at Methodist Hospital; and Graham Serjeant, director of the Medical Research Counsel Laboratory, University of the West Indies, Jamaica. They all remembered their experiences with him and what he had meant to them as mentor, researcher, clinician, and human being. Those present were reminded that Diggs kept a commonplace book, the one he had started as a medical student at Hopkins, which contained the aphorisms and sayings of poets and scientists; when taken together, these items that he recorded and saved probably came as close as any document could to capturing the landscape of his personality.[62] Ann Bell announced the "cherished honor" of organizing all of Diggs's writings on sickle cell with the help of Daniel Brookoff and Walter Diggs. "With these future plans," she said, "we want to make available to anyone interested in sickle cell disease the theories, ideas, and knowledge of this dedicated, compassionate, studious, kind and remarkable physician—Lemuel Whitley Diggs."[63]

Conclusion
A Life Well Lived

For most of his career, Lemuel Whitley Diggs worked on sickle cell anemia, a disorder that was invisible to the people who were most likely to suffer from it, that interested relatively few researchers, and for which almost no research funding was available. As a physician and a southerner, he understood the complexity and seriousness of the problems plaguing the South, especially racism and its ability to disadvantage a people and a country as well as to discourage genuine research. Yet, curing the disease, the one that afflicted the body and the one afflicting society, was his goal. His answer was to humanize the problem by giving as precise a scientific definition as possible and to both humanize the disease faced by sufferers and replace the cultural conception of the disease with certain scientific knowledge. He was never under any illusion that the task would be simple or the answer easy to find. He had a paramount sense of individual responsibility and of social order throughout his life. The problems he saw in society could only be solved by everyone working together within the social context until a better order could be found.

Early in his life, Diggs knew that he wanted to be the best physician possible, and he strove to live the best life he could. As a physician, he personified the traditional maxim that, if one learns a single disease well, one knows medicine well. His teachers at John Hopkins University, following in the tradition of William Osler, inspired him to apply the full weight of his energy to science and medicine and to minimize his nonscientific interests. Diggs believed that any problem could be solved and society improved by a rational method, by "using one's head." He believed this whether he was considering a scientific, a practical, or a spiritual question. At the same time, he was an active skeptic who loved to debate, and he was willing to debate unpopular subjects, from the membership of black physicians in the Memphis and Shelby County Medical Society to the vicissitudes of national healthcare policy. He began his life with a pledge to himself—or rather, to humanity—to be the best man he could be, "clean, strong, happy, honest, truthful and hard working," the best doctor and teacher of internal medicine, and thorough in all he undertook. His older son, Walter, recalled: "He was never motivated by money. He was more interested in being a skeptic. Someone who questioned things to make them clearer and truer. A seeker after knowledge. Then, because he was a very scientific person, he decided what he wanted to believe and then he practiced that."[1]

Diggs also believed in a balanced life, one in which the demands of his professional life could be counterbalanced by his private life; he aimed "to use his time better, allowing space for relaxation, physical exercise, and social enjoyment."[2] He was never interested in social activities; his "country club" was the garden that he cultivated on his farm in Whitehaven, and later in Cordova. His wife, Beatrice Moshier, was his equal partner. Along with being the best physician he could be, he wanted "the love of a real woman," which he found in her. They had four children together; she typed and edited his work and accompanied him on many of his professional trips as projectionist and organizer. They both enjoyed gardening. He was a gentleman farmer, a throwback in some sense to the Colonial idea of the farmer as the perfect citizen. Beatrice kept a cow at one time, which she milked. According to Walter Diggs, "She loved milk, boiled fresh cow's milk."[3] The garden was always a family occupation, and she was passionate about it. Their partnership involved both personal and professional activities, remaining rich and strong for many decades.

Once Diggs arrived in Memphis, he became aware of the unusually high number of sickle cell sufferers. His decision to investigate sickle cell was both a medical and a political one. He would make the same decision again in the creation of the blood bank and in counseling against using race in admitting patients to St. Jude Children's Research Hospital. The threads of sickle cell and racism run through Diggs's professional life. He was the first to posit that clumps of sickled red cells, "log jams" as he put it, were the cause of the excruciating pain characterizing "crisis" in patients. He also saw the sickle cell trait as a discrete entity, separate from the full-blown disease, and argued that patients with the trait should not be included in research because their condition was compatible with normal life and not to be confused with the disease itself. As a white physician in Memphis endeavoring to conduct serious research into sickle cell, he sought and earned the trust of many in the black community.

Diggs created the first sickle cell center in the United States in 1958 with minimal local support; it expanded in 1971 with the availability of federal funding. As Diggs envisioned it, the center would provide a venue for the kind of research he wanted to conduct in order to find relief and possibly a cure. In his lifetime, the simplest remedies remained the best for treating the disease. Although there was progress in understanding, the puzzle of the disease never yielded to Diggs's determined attempts to solve it. Diggs also opened the first blood bank in the South, supported technology as a necessary component of the medical curriculum, and helped found and organize St. Jude Children's Research Hospital. Not the least of his accomplishments was as an educator of thousands of students and residents, of colleagues in hundreds of off-campus classes, and of medical professionals by means of his publications.

Diggs recognized that racism was an intractable and complex problem that could not be solved easily, and least of all by confrontation. Instead, he addressed the problem through his research into all aspects of sickle cell disease and by ignoring Jim Crow strictures when they were incompatible with medical knowledge. He continued to educate his patients even after being told by his dean, "We don't teach them." He hired a black medical technician and stood by him when a white woman complained that a "nigger" was drawing blood from her. The Memphis police commissioner complained, but Diggs ignored him and nothing came of the matter. He was expected to segregate blood units in the blood bank; he disregarded the policy when it contradicted medical understanding, offering blood across color lines with the informed permission of the patients. During the challenging days of the civil rights movement, he publicly called for an end to segregated access to the public library and the zoo in Memphis, rebuked a white supremacist seeking medical justification for the biological separation of the races, and advocated for the acceptance of black physicians into the Memphis and Shelby County Medical Society.

In keeping with his Methodist upbringing, Diggs gave high priority to service to his profession and to his country. Politically he was a moderate throughout his life: he encountered the problem of racism on a daily basis but avoided dividing his efforts by focusing on only the most important problem at hand. The concept of a man that he articulated for himself while growing up was that of acting honorably and civilly. It was never in his nature to speak out or to rebel against social illness, but rather to recognize the intractability of the problem and to work steadily to change it. While he could not change the prejudices around him, he could act differently himself by closing the door when he wanted to educate his black patients about sickle cell and other illnesses, and ignore the policy to segregate blood units.

Diggs was an independent thinker who believed that he should rely on the brains that God had given him to solve all problems, including spiritual ones. His early experiences in family religious debates, combined with his own sense of doubt, led him to move away from the zeal of his family's Methodist faith, and their desire that he become a minister, to abiding commitments to medicine and the Unitarian faith. He always sought a single, integrated truth in life and in science. His skepticism functioned to question accepted beliefs until the facts merged to form knowledge, and then he would practice that knowledge. He was inclusive of all people, regardless of their religion, preferring to treat his staff and others around him as a team. He rejected the "plantation mentality," common at medical centers at the time, in how both patients and medical staff were treated.[4]

The doctor-patient relationship, based on trust and mutual respect, lay at the heart of Diggs's treatment of the ills of his patients and those of society. His interest in people was beneficent and deliberate. Diggs was animated by the belief that his task was to make life better for others. He wanted to uplift his country, and applying intellectual skills to finding the solution to the most intractable problems was his way to achieve that goal.

Even though Diggs's lifelong efforts to find a cure for sickle cell anemia remained unsuccessful—and to date a cure still has not been found—his accomplishments in research, blood-banking, helping to found a major hospital, and promoting the dignity and rights of individuals of all races embodied the timeless qualities of a model physician. His ideals continue to resonate and inspire those who carry on his noble-hearted work.

Notes

Introduction

Epigraph: Diggs, Lemuel W. Notebook. 1924. The Lemuel W. Diggs Collection, The University of Tennessee Health Sciences Historical Collections, Memphis, TN. See page 24 for epigraph.

1. L. W. Diggs, "Notebook of Collected Sayings," 1924. There are two handwritten commonplace books containing aphorisms and sayings that Diggs considered most meaningful for his worldview or for the profession of medicine. The notebooks can be found in the Lemuel W. Diggs Collection, University of Tennessee Health Sciences Historical Collections, Memphis.

2. Diggs, *First Portion,* audio recording with no date found in: The Lemuel W. Diggs Collection, Manuscript Collection, The University of Tennessee Health Sciences Historical Collections.

3. In the absence of reliable statistics, the ratio of black to white patients is anecdotal from several sources. See also Frank D. Smyth, "A Golden Opportunity for the University of Tennessee Medical College." *Memphis Medical Journal* 1, (1924): 214–18.

4. Lloyd M. Graves, "The Public Health Situation in Memphis," *Memphis Medical Journal* (March 1929): 56–59; Marvin L. Graves, "The Negro a Menace to the Health of the White Race," *Southern Medical Journal* 19, no. 4 (1916): 407–13; Joe Adcock and Cynthia Adcock, "Houston's Hospitals: The Smell of Charity," *Nation* 200, no. 1 (1965): 5–8. A first-hand account of mistreatment in the John Gaston Hospital can be found in: D'Army Bailey with Roger R. Easson. *The Education of a Black Radical: A Southern Civil Rights Activist's Journey, 1959–1964,* foreword by Nikki Giavonni. Baton Rouge: Louisiana State University Press, 2009.

5. G. Wayne Dowdy and Edward Hull Crump, *Mayor Crump Don't Like It: Machine Politics in Memphis* (Jackson: University Press of Mississippi, 2006), 89–90, 111.

6. Marcus J. Stewart, William Thomas Black, and Mildred Hicks, eds., *History of Medicine in Memphis* (Memphis: Memphis and Shelby County Medical Society, 1971), 407, 261–62.

7. Eric Hoffer, *The True Believer: Thoughts on the Nature of Mass Movements* (1951; rpt. New York: Harper Perennial, 2002), 8.

Chapter 1

Epigraph: Diggs, Lemuel W. Notebook. 1924. The Lemuel W. Diggs Collection, The University of Tennessee Health Sciences Historical Collections, Memphis, TN.

1. L. W. Diggs, "Health Care and Human Rights," audio recording, Lemuel W. Diggs Collection; Richard Nollan, interview with Walter Diggs, Memphis, June 13, 2008.

2. David M. Kennedy, *Over Here: The First World War and American Society* (New York: Oxford University Press, 2004).

3. James Edward Scanlon, *Randolph-Macon College: A Southern History, 1825–1967* (Charlottesville: University Press of Virginia, 1983).

4. Lemuel W. Diggs Collection, folder LWD 001-1. Also see Literary Societies of Randolph-Macon College, *The Yellow Jacket* (Ashland, VA: Randolph-Macon College, 1921), and *The Yellow Jacket Annual* (Ashland, VA: Randolph-Macon College, 1920).

5. Scanlon, *Randolph-Macon College*, 287–321.

6. Lemuel W. Diggs Collection, Folder LWD 001-1, contains numerous photos of Diggs's early years, and includes a clipping of a debating victory naming Diggs on the opposing side over a rival school.

7. The Literary Societies of Randolph-Macon College. *The Yellow Jacket*. Vol. XXIX. Ashland, VA: Randolph-Macon College, 1921. See page 73 for quotation.

8. *Records of the Johns Hopkins University School of Medicine,* Johns Hopkins University, Baltimore, MD. See Diggs's admission application (undated); JHU Registrar [G. J. Coy] to Diggs, May 25, 1922; and Diggs's letter to G. J. Coy, May 28, 1922.

9. Ibid.; Literary Societies of Randolph-Macon College, *The Yellow Jacket*, 1922.

10. Abraham Flexner, Henry S. Pritchett, and Carnegie Foundation for the Advancement of Teaching, *Medical Education in the United States and Canada: A Report to the Carnegie Foundation for the Advancement of Teaching* (New York City, 1910).

11. "The History of Johns Hopkins Medicine," www.hopkinsmedicine. org/about/history/; Harry F. Dowling, *City Hospitals: The Undercare of the Underprivileged* (Cambridge, MA: Harvard University Press, 1982), 115.

12. Letter from the Dean to L. W. Diggs, June 15, 1922 found in: *Records of the Johns Hopkins University School of Medicine,* Johns Hopkins University, Baltimore, MD.

13. Kenneth M. Ludmerer, *Time to Heal: American Medical Education from the Turn of the Century to the Era of Managed Care* (Oxford, UK: Oxford University Press, 1999), 72.

14. L. W. Diggs, by an anonymous interviewer, audio recording, 1976. The audio recording can be found in: Johns Hopkins Medical Institutions. Alan Mason Chesney Medical Archives. Baltimore, MD.

15. William G. Rothstein, *American Medical Schools and the Practice of Medicine* (New York: Oxford University Press, 1987), 170; Edward C. Atwater, "'Making Fewer Mistakes', A History of Students and Patients," *Bulletin of the History of Medicine* 57, (1987): 165–87, see especially 180.

16. Maxwell M. Wintrobe, ed., *Blood, Pure and Eloquent: A Story of Discovery, of People, and of Ideas* (New York: McGraw-Hill Book Co., 1980).

17. Simon D. Feldman and Alfred I. Tauber, "Sickle Cell Anemia: Reexamining the First 'Molecular Disease,'" *Bulletin of the History of Medicine* 71, no. 4 (1997): 623–50.

18. Nollan, interview with Walter Diggs, 2008.

19. Elinor Bluemel, *Florence Sabin: Colorado Woman of the Century* (Boulder: University of Colorado Press, 1959).

20. Interview with L. W. Diggs, 1976, anonymous interviewer. Audio recording found in the "Collection Johns Hopkins University School of Medicine—Records of the Johns Hopkins School of Medicine," Baltimore, MD.

21. "Art as Applied to Medicine," Johns Hopkins Medicine, accessed July 14, 2015, www.hopkinsmedicine.org/about/history/history7.html; Wintrobe, ed., *Blood, Pure and Eloquent,* 334.

22. James Edward Hamner, *The University of Tennessee, Memphis 75th Anniversary: Medical Accomplishments* (Memphis: University of Tennessee, 1986), 74.

23. Interview with L. W. Diggs by an anonymous interviewer, recorded 1976. The audio recording of this interview can be found in: Johns Hopkins Medical Institutions. Alan Mason Chesney Medical Archives. Baltimore, MD.

24. Lemuel W. Diggs Collection, folder LWD 001-711.

25. Ibid., folder LWD 001-1.

26. Jules Cohen and Robert J. Joynt, eds., *The University of Rochester Medical Center: Teaching, Discovering, Caring: Seventy-Five Years of Achievement, 1925–2000* (Rochester, NY: University of Rochester Press, 2000), 192.

27. Nollan, interview with Diggs, June 13, 2008.

28. Lemuel W. Diggs Collection, folder LDW 001-7-12.

29. L. W. Diggs, "Dr. George Hoyt Whipple," *Johns Hopkins Medical Journal* 139, no. 5 (November 1976): 196–200. See page 199 for quotation.

30. *Legenda,* Wellesley College yearbook, 1926.

31. Wintrobe, ed., *Blood, Pure and Eloquent;* Cohen and Joynt, eds., *The University of Rochester Medical Center;* Walter Diggs interview by Richard Nollan.

32. Diggs, "Dr. George Hoyt Whipple," 196–200. See page 199 for quotation.

33. Lemuel W. Diggs Collection, folder LWD 001-1.

34. Diggs, "Dr. George Hoyt Whipple," 196–200. See page 197 for quotation.

35. Lemuel W. Diggs Collection, folder 001-9-12.

36. Keith Wailoo, *Dying in the City of the Blues: Sickle Cell Anemia and the Politics of Race and Health* (Chapel Hill: University of North Carolina Press, 2001), 338; Frieda S. Robscheit-Robbins and George H. Whipple, "Blood Regeneration in Severe Anemia: A Liver Fraction Potent in Pernicious Anemia Fed Alone and Combined with Whole Liver, Liver Ash and Fresh Bile," *Journal of Experimental Medicine* 49, no. 2 (1929): 215–27.

37. Alfred Paul Kraus, "A Reminiscent Journey with . . . Lemuel Whitley Diggs, M.D.," *Tennessee Medical Alumnus* (Spring 1968): 2.

38. O. W. Hyman, "Notes on the Development of the Medical Units, University of Tennessee, Strictly through the Eyes and Prejudices of O. W. Hyman," typescript manuscript in: Simon Rulin Bruesch Collection, folder 051-32, University of Tennessee Health Sciences Library Historical Collections. This history of the institution was written around 1974 by one of the University of Tennessee Medical Unit's most influential figures.

39. Jerry Francisco, MD. Interview with Richard Nollan, Memphis, 2011.

40. Rothstein, *American Medical Schools,* 158.

41. Lemuel W. Diggs Collection, folder 002-6-1.

42. Herman G. Weiskotten, Alphonse M. Schwitalla, William D. Cutter, and Hamilton H. Anderson, *Medical Education in the United States 1934–1939* (Chicago: American Medical Association, 1940), 58.

Chapter 2

Epigraph: From Diggs, Notebook, 1924. The quotation is also found in William Osler, *A Way of Life: An Address Delivered to Yale Students, Sunday Evening, April 20th, 1913* (Springfield, IL: Thomas, 1969).

1. Hamner, *University of Tennessee, Memphis 75th Anniversary,* 35. See also Mary Roth Walsh, *Doctors Wanted: No Women Need Apply: Sexual Barriers in the Medical Profession, 1835–1975* (New Haven, CT: Yale University Press, 1979).

2. Hamner, *University of Tennessee, Memphis 75th Anniversary;* Stewart, Black, and Hicks, eds., *History of Medicine in Memphis,* 407; James Summerville, *Nashville Medicine: A History* (Dallas, TX: Taylor Publishing Co., 1999), 35.

3. Diggs, "Dr. George Hoyt Whipple," 196–200.

4. Roger Biles, *Memphis in the Great Depression* (Knoxville: University of Tennessee Press, 1986), 174.

5. Douglas W. Cupples, "Memphis Confederates: The Civil War and its Aftermath," PhD dissertation, University of Memphis, 1995; Douglas W. Cupples, "A Short Medical History of Memphis, Tennessee." Presentation, Tennessee Conference of Historians, Chattanooga, TN, September 2, 2011.

6. Stewart, Black, and Hicks, eds., *History of Medicine in Memphis,* 407, 19–44; Patricia M. LaPointe, *From Saddlebags to Science: A Century of Health Care in Memphis, 1830–1930* (Memphis: Health Sciences Museum Foundation of the Memphis and Shelby County Medical Society Auxiliary, 1984), 124.

7. LaPointe, From Saddlebags to Science, 31.

8. G. Wayne Dowdy, *A Brief History of Memphis* (Charleston, SC: History Press, 2011), 120, 57–58.

9. Biles, *Memphis in the Great Depression,* 174, 50.

10. Hamner, *University of Tennessee, Memphis 75th Anniversary;* Biles, *Memphis in the Great Depression,* 174; Dowdy and Crump, *Mayor Crump Don't Like It.*

11. Dowdy and Crump, *Mayor Crump Don't Like It,* 10–11, 66–67.

12. Biles, *Memphis in the Great Depression,* 174; see table, "Origins of Memphis Population by State of Birth, 1930," 30.

13. Roger Biles, "The Persistence of the Past: Memphis in the Great Depression," *Journal of Southern History* 52, no. 2 (1986): 183, 185.

14. Gerald M. Capers Jr., *The Biography of a River Town: Memphis: Its Heroic Age* (Memphis, TN: Burke's Store, 1966; rpt. 2003), 119–20, 206–7. Also see Allison Collis Greene, *No Depression in Heaven: Religion and Economic Crisis in Memphis and the Delta, 1929–1941* (Ann Arbor, MI: ProQuest, 2010).

15. Greene, *No Depression in Heaven,* 2010. See page 34 for quote.

16. Alice Diggs, interview by Richard Nollan, October 26, 2011, audio file.

17. Walter Diggs, interview by Richard Nollan, 2008.

18. Lemuel W. Diggs Collection, photographs, folder 001-01.

19. Walter Diggs, interview by Richard Nollan, 2008; Alice Diggs, interview by Richard Nollan, 2011.

20. Thomas H. Baker, *The Memphis Commercial Appeal: The History of a Southern Newspaper* (Baton Rouge: Louisiana State University Press, 1971), 336.

21. Biles, "The Persistence of the Past," 183, 186.

22. Hamner, *University of Tennessee, Memphis 75th Anniversary,* 85.

23. Biles, "The Persistence of the Past," 183, 187.

24. Ludmerer, *Time to Heal*; Kathryn Montgomery, *How Doctors Think: Clinical Judgment and the Practice of Medicine* (New York: Oxford University Press, 2006).

25. Walter Diggs, "LW Diggs Heroes," email message to author, September 25, 2008.

26. Michael Bliss, *William Osler: A Life in Medicine* (Oxford: Oxford University Press, 1999), 1. See page 268; Harvey Cushing, *The Life of Sir William Osler* (London: Oxford University Press, 1940); "William Osler—Biography," www.medicalarchives.jhmi.edu/osler/biography.htm.

27. Walter Diggs, email to author, September 25, 2008, 1.

28. "Blood picture" is a generally used phrase in the language of this time that refers to the microscopic observations of the percentage of blood cells and their condition. Later the phrase would become more metaphorical as laboratory test results were included as part of the blood analysis.

29. Thelma Tracy Mabry and L. W. Diggs, *History of Medicine in Memphis: Interview with Dr. Lemuel Whitley Diggs* (Memphis: Oral History Research Office, Memphis State University, 1984).

30. Lemuel W. Diggs Collection, autobiographical writings, folder 001-1-13.

31. The concept of scientific objectivity, which was a highly esteemed hallmark of scientific thinking, was one that Diggs also aspired to maintain in his thinking. A recent work that illustrates this is: Lorraine Daston and Peter Galison, *Objectivity* (New York: Zone Books, 2007).

32. Smythe, "A Golden Opportunity," 216.

33. Kraus, "A Reminiscent Journey," 2.

34. Ibid.

35. L. W. Diggs, "The Sickle Cell Center in Memphis," File Card Index, *The Press-Scimitar* Morgue File, University of Memphis, Ned McWherter Library, Special Collections, file 80145, p. 1–2.

36. Vivien Thomas, *Partners of the Heart* (Philadelphia: University of Pennsylvania Press, 1985), 245; W. Michael Byrd and Linda A. Clayton, *An American Health Dilemma: Race, Medicine, and Health Care in the United States: 1900–2000* (New York: Routledge, 2002).

37. Paul Starr, *The Social Transformation of American Medicine: The Rise of a Sovereign Profession and the Making of a Vast Industry* (New York: Basic Books, Inc., 1982), 121. For a broader description, see Rothstein, *American Medical Schools.*

38. Mabry and Diggs, *History of Medicine in Memphis,* 1.

39. Julian M. Ruffin and David T. Smith, "The Treatment of Pellagra with Certain Preparations of Liver," *American Journal of the Medical Science* 187, no. 4 (1934): 512–20.

40. Orren W. Hyman. "Notes on the Development of the Medical Units, University of Tennessee." [Sweetwater, Tenn.], typescript manuscript located in: Simon Rulin Bruesch Collection, folder 051-32, University of Tennessee Health Sciences Library Historical Collections.

41. Dr. Bruesch's notes about the history of pathology, Simon R. Bruesch Collection, folder 024-5.

42. L. W. Diggs, "Clinical Pathology," in Stewart, Black, and Hicks, eds., *History of Medicine in Memphis,* 240.

43. Smythe, "A Golden Opportunity," 216.

44. Flexner, Pritchett, and Carnegie Foundation, *Medical Education in the United States and Canada*, 346.

45. Dowling, *City Hospitals*, 153.

46. Mabry and Diggs, *History of Medicine in Memphis*, 6–7.

47. Travis Winsor and George E. Burch, "Sickle Cell Anemia: A Great Masquerader," *Journal of the American Medical Association* 129 (1947): 793–96; L. W. Diggs, H. N. Pulliam, and J. C. King, "Bone Changes in Sickle Cell Anemia," *Southern Medical Journal* 30, no. 3 (1937): 258.

48. Lemuel W. Diggs, Sickle Cell Notebook B, Lemuel W. Diggs Collection, p. b73 [79].

49. Mabry and Diggs, *History of Medicine in Memphis*.

50. Lemuel W. Diggs Collection, folder 001-7-13.

51. Paul Reznikof, "Anemia," in *A Text-Book of Medicine by American Authors* (Philadelphia: W. B. Saunders Co., 1927), 921–26; A. Piney, *Diseases of the Blood*, 2nd ed. (Philadelphia: P. Blakiston's Son & Co. Inc., 1932); A. Piney and Stanley Wyard, *Clinical Atlas of Blood Diseases*, 2nd. ed. (Philadelphia: P. Blakiston's Son & Co. Inc., 1932).

52. Hans Hirschfeld, *Lehrbuch der Blutkrankheiten für Artze und Studierende*, 2nd ed. (Leipzig: Verlag von Johann Ambrosius Barth, 1928); Otto Naegeli, *Blutkrankheiten und Blutdiagnostik: Lehrbuch der Klinischen Hämatolgie* (Berlin: Verlag von Julius Springer, 1931).

53. American Medical Association and National Library of Medicine, *Quarterly Cumulative Index Medicus* (Chicago: n.p., 1927–56).

54. Mabry and Diggs, *History of Medicine in Memphis*.

55. The note can be found in the bound volume marked 1929-4 of *The L. W. Diggs, M.D. Sickle Cell Literature Collection: 1910–1970*, compiled by Lemuel W. Diggs with assistance of the Bluff City Medical and Pharmaceutical Auxiliary (Memphis: n.p., 1981), located in the University of Tennessee Health Sciences Historical Collections. No page numbers. The article commented on was: V. P. Sydenstricker, "Sickle-Cell Anemia," *Medical Clinics of North America*, 12 (1929): 1451–57.

56. J. B. Herrick, "Peculiar Elongated and Sickle-Shaped Red Blood Corpuscles in a Case of Severe Anemia," *Archives of Internal Medicine* 5 (1910): 517, 518. Similar sickle cells had been described in animal blood as early as 1840; see C. Lockard Conley, "Sickle-Cell Anemia—the First Molecular Disease," in Wintrobe, ed., *Blood, Pure and Eloquent*, 320.

57. B. E. Washburn, "Peculiar Elongated and Sickle-Shaped Red Blood Corpuscles in a Case of Severe Anemia," *Virginia Medical Semi-Monthly* 15 (1911): 490–93.

58. Jerome E. Cook and Jerome Meyer, "Peculiar Elongated and Sickle-Shaped Red Blood Corpuscles in a Case of Severe Anemia." *Archives of Internal Medicine* 16 (1915): 644–51.

59. Victor E. Emmel, "A Study of the Erythrocytes in a Case of Severe Anemia with Elongated and Sickle-Shaped Red Blood Corpuscles," *Archive of Internal Medicine* 20 (1917): 586–98. The blood picture would become not only a means of diagnosis, but also of establishing heredity.

60. John G. Huck, "Sickle Cell Anemia," *Johns Hopkins Hospital Bulletin* 34 (1923): 335–44.

61. V. R. Mason, "Sickle-Cell Anemia," *Journal of the American Medical Association* 79 (1922): 1318–22.

62. Ibid.

63. V. P. Sydenstricker, W. A. Mulherin, and R. W. Houseal, "Sickle Cell Anemia: Report of Two Cases in Children, with Necropsy in One Case," *Archives of Pediatrics* 40 (1923): 154.

64. Ibid.; Virgil P. Sydenstricker, "Sickle Cell Anemia." *Southern Medical Journal* 17 (1924): 177–83. In *Dying in the City of the Blues* (78), Wailoo argues that the significance of focusing on sickle cell disease as a Mendelian disease is that only one parent with the trait is needed in order to transmit the disease to the offspring. A racist, for whom sickle cell is considered a "black" disease, could easily envision its being transferred from the black to the white race through miscegenation.

65. Feldman and Tauber, "Sickle Cell Anemia," 633.

66. J. F. Hamilton, "A Case of Sickle Cell Anemia." *Memphis Medical Journal* 2, no. 11 (1925): 253–55.

67. Memphis General Hospital, *Report of Patients Discharged during the Month of April 1927: Principal Diseases* (Memphis: Memphis City Hospital, 1927).

68. Wailoo, *Dying in the City of the Blues,* chap. 1; Alfred P. Kraus, Lorraine Kraus, and Jim Gibb Johnson, "Oral Interview with Alfred P. and Lorraine Kraus," Oral History, University of Tennessee Health Science Center Oral History Project, Memphis, p. 1 and 3; T. L. Savitt, "The Invisible Malady: Sickle Cell Anemia in America, 1910–1970," *Journal of the National Medical Association* 73, no. 8 (August 1981): 739–46.

69. Adcock and Adcock, "Houston's Hospitals," 8; Dowling, *City Hospitals*; Vanessa Northington Gamble, "Under the Shadow of Tuskegee: African Americans and Health Care," *American Journal of Public Health* 87, no. 11 (1997): 1773–78.

70. Walter Diggs, interview by Richard Nollan, June 13, 2008, audio file.

71. Ludmerer, *Time to Heal*; Starr, *Social Transformation of American Medicine.*

72. Graves, "The Negro a Menace," 407–13.

73. Ibid., 412.

74. Robert A. Divine et al., *The American Story,* 3rd ed. (New York: Pearson Longman, 2007), 665–66.

75. Graves, "The Public Health Situation in Memphis," 59.

76. Jerry Francisco, interview by Richard Nollan, 2011, audio file.

77. Montgomery, *How Doctors Think*; Kathryn Montgomery Hunter, *Doctors' Stories: The Narrative Structure of Medical Knowledge* (Princeton, NJ: Princeton University Press, 1991).

78. L. W. Diggs, "The Blood Picture in Sickle Cell Anemia," *Southern Medical Journal* 25 (1932): 615–20.

79. Ibid., 615.

80. Von Jaksch's anemia is characterized by anemia, high white cell count, an enlarged spleen, and fever. By 1925 it was included under the heading of "thalassemia." See D. J. Weatherall, "Toward an Understanding of the Molecular

Biology of Some Common Inherited Anemias: The Story of Thalassemia," in Wintrobe, ed., *Blood, Pure and Eloquent,* 375–76. For more on the quotation at the end of the paragraph, see Diggs, "The Blood Picture in Sickle Cell Anemia," 617.

81. Harry C. Schmeisser and J. L. Scianni, "Art as Applied to Medicine," *Journal of the Tennessee Medical Association* 19 (1926–27): 311–15; H. C. Schmeisser, J. V. Caltagirone, and J. L. Scianni, "Graphic Art and Its Application to the Teaching of Medicine: Animated Film," *Southern Medical Journal* 25 (1932): 886–88; Max Brödel, "The Origin, Growth, and Future of Medical Illustration at the Johns Hopkins Hospital and Medical School," *Johns Hopkins Hospital Bulletin* 26 (1915): 184–90; Daston and Galison, *Objectivity.*

82. Lynn Dumenil, *Modern Temper: American Culture and Society in the 1920s* (New York: Hill and Wang, 1995). Walter Diggs, interview by Richard Nollan, audio file.

83. E. C. Smith, "A Case of Malaria with a Blood Picture Suggestive of Splenic Anaemia," *West African Medical Journal* 4 (1932): 69.

84. Diggs, "Dr. George Hoyt Whipple," 196–200.

85. E. C. Smith, "Letter to the Editor," *West African Medical Journal* (June 21, 1933), clipping found in in a bound volume marked "Medical Publications.

86. Mabry and Diggs, *History of Medicine in Memphis.*

87. L. W. Diggs and R. E. Ching, "Pathology of Sickle-Cell Anemia," *Southern Medical Journal* 27 (1934): 340.

88. R. E. Ching and L. W. Diggs, "Splenectomy in Sickle-Cell Anemia; Report of a Case with Necropsy in an Adult on Whom Splenectomy Was Attempted," *Archives of Internal Medicine* 51 (1933): 101. Dr. Ching was a faculty member in the Pathology Department during these years, but little is know about his time at the University of Tennessee.

89. Mabry and Diggs, *History of Medicine in Memphis,* 14.

90. Diggs, "Clinical Pathology," 253–54.

91. Ching and Diggs, "Splenectomy in Sickle-Cell Anemia," 100–11.

92. L. W. Diggs, "Siderofibrosis of the Spleen in Sickle Cell Anemia," *Journal of the American Medical Association* 104 (1935): 538–41. See page 541 for quotation.

93. Thelma Tracy Mabry and L. W. Diggs, *History of Medicine in Memphis: Interview with Dr. Lemuel Whitley Diggs,* (Memphis, Tenn.: Oral History Research Office, Memphis State University, 1984). See page 15 for quotation.

94. Ibid, page 15.

95. Ibid, page 15.

96. Ibid, page 15.

97. O. W. Hyman, "The Tennessee Four-Quarter Plan," *Journal of the Association of American Medical Colleges* 4 (1929): 300–307; L. W. Diggs, "The Four-Quarter System at the University of Tennessee," *Southern Medical Journal* 29, no. 10 (1936): 1014–20; O. W. Hyman, "The Influence of Recent Changes in the Distribution of Physicians upon the Conditions of Medical Practice in Tennessee," *Memphis Medical Journal* 9 (1932): 93–96. Hyman was concerned about the steadily declining numbers of physicians working in rural Tennessee communities. He believed that the four-quarter system would make medical education affordable to lower-income students and that 70 percent of these students would return to their home communities after graduation. If so, he

reasoned, the four-quarter system would assist lower-income men to seek a medical degree and help reverse the demographic shift of doctors from the countryside to the city.

98. Simon R. Bruesch Collection, folder 024-05, p. 8.

99. L. W. Diggs and Ernestine T. Flowers, *"The Socio-Economic Problems in Sickle Cell Anemia,"* 1976, See manuscript page 2 for quotation. This typescript manuscript is located in a bound volume of miscellaneous publication in: L. W. Diggs Collection, University of Tennessee Health Sciences Historical Collections.

100. Diggs and Flowers, *The Socio-Economic Problems in Sickle Cell Anemia.*

101. Perhaps the Tuskegee Project is the starkest reminder of the extent of medical racism at the time. The longest nontherapeutic medical project began in 1932 in Alabama and continued to 1972. See Susan Reverby, *Examining Tuskegee: The Infamous Syphilis Study and its Legacy* (Chapel Hill: University of North Carolina Press, 2009).

102. Susan E. Lederer, *Subjected to Science: Human Experimentation in America before the Second World War* (Baltimore: Johns Hopkins University Press, 1995), 111.

103. I. A. McSwani, "Some of the Opposing Forces to Rational Therapeutics," *Memphis Medical Monthly* 25, no. 9 (1905): 468.

104. J. Wasserman, M. A. Flannery, and J. M. Clair, "Raising the Ivory Tower: The Production of Knowledge and Distrust of Medicine among African Americans," *Journal of Medical Ethics* 33, no. 3 (Mar 2007): 177–80.

Chapter 3

Epigraph: Diggs. Notebook. 1924.

1. Lemuel W. Diggs Collection, letter from Diggs to W. E. Quick, October 11, 1937, folder 002-6-4.

2. Nollan, interview with Diggs, 2011.

3. Biles, *Memphis in the Great Depression,* 69.

4. Biles, "The Persistence of the Past," 202.

5. Diggs, "Clinical Pathology," 246.

6. Ibid.

7. Ibid.

8. Hyman, "The Tennessee Four-Quarter Plan," 302.

9. Hyman, "The Influence of Recent Changes in the Distribution of Physicians," 94.

10. Ludmerer, *Time to Heal,* 99.

11. Diggs, "The Four-Quarter System," 1018.

12. Ludmerer, *Time to Heal,* 100.

13. Ibid., 100–101.

14. L. W. Diggs, "The Training of Medical Technologists as a Function of the Medical School," *Southern Medical Journal* 35 (1942): 1104–7.

15. See Bruesch's Pathology Department notes in Simon R. Bruesch Collection, folders 024-4 and 024-5.

16. Diggs, "Clinical Pathology," 255–64. Diggs was an academic researcher with a habit of reviewing all relevant medical literature in all questions that

interested him. See J. R. Hess and P. J. Schmidt, "The First Blood Banker: Oswald Hope Robertson," *Transfusion* 40, no. 1 (2000): 110–13.

17. Sarah E. Chinn, *Technology and the Logic of American Racism: A Cultural History of the Body as Evidence* (London: Continuum, 2000) 233; Louis Diamond, "A History of Blood Transfusion," in Wintrobe, ed., *Blood, Pure and Eloquent,* 659–88.

18. Douglas Starr, *Blood: An Epic History of Medicine and Commerce* (New York: Alfred A. Knopf, 1998); Susan E. Lederer, *Flesh and Blood: Organ Transplantation and Blood Transfusion in 20th Century America* (Oxford: Oxford University Press, 2008); L. K. Diamond, "History of Blood Banking in the United States," *JAMA: The Journal of the American Medical Association* 193 (1965): 40–44.

19. Diamond, Louis, "A History of Blood Transfusion," in *Blood, Pure and Eloquent: A Story of Discovery, of People, and of Ideas,* edited by Wintrobe, Maxwell M., 659–88 (New York: McGraw-Hill Book Co., 1980). See page 672.

20. Diamond, "A History of Blood Transfusion," 659–88.

21. Ibid.; Louis K. Diamond, "The Story of Our Blood Groups," in Wintrobe, ed., *Blood, Pure and Eloquent,* 691–717.

22. Diamond, "A History of Blood Transfusion," 677–78.

23. S. B. Moore, "A Brief History of the Early Years of Blood Transfusion at the Mayo Clinic: The First Blood Bank in the United States (1935)," *Transfusion Medicine Reviews* 19, no. 3 (2005): 241–45.

24. M. Telischi, "Evolution of Cook County Hospital Blood Bank," *Transfusion* 14, no. 6 (1974): 623–28.

25. Ann Bell, "Portrait of L. W. Diggs, M.D.," Tennessee Association of Blood Banks, accessed October 6, 2007, www.tabbonline.org/LW_Diggs_portrait.html.

26. [L. W. Diggs], *Memorandum to the John Gaston Hospital Medical Board,* unpublished memorandum in: L. W. Diggs Collection, University of Tennessee Health Sciences Historical Collections, folder 002-06.

27. L. W. Diggs, "First Portion," audio file, n.d., University of Tennessee Health Sciences Historical Collections. This recording was probably made in anticipation of his acceptance of the Virginian of the Year Award in 1978.

28. Ann Bell in discussion with the author, September 24, 2007.

29. Diggs, L. W., "Clinical Pathology," in *History of Medicine in Memphis,* edited by Stewart, Marcus J., William Thomas Black, and Mildred Hicks, 239–64, (Memphis: Memphis and Shelby County Medical Society, 1971).

30. Ibid. See page 259 for quotation.

31. *Memorandum to the John Gaston Hospital Medical Board.*

32. Diggs, "Clinical Pathology," 239–64.

33. Ibid.

34. L. W. Diggs and Alice Jean Keith, "Problems in Blood Banking," *American Journal of Clinical Pathology* 9, no. 6 (1939): 594.

35. Reuben L. Kahn, *The Kahn Test—A Practical Guide* (New York: Williams and Wilkins Co., 1928).

36. H. D. Packer, "Forty-five Years against Syphilis in Memphis—Success or Failure?" *Journal of the Tennessee Medical Association* 77, no. 2 (1984): 75–79.

37. Keith Wailoo, *Drawing Blood: Technology and Disease Identity in Twentieth-Century America* (Baltimore: Johns Hopkins University Press, 1997). See page 136 for quotation.

38. Waldemar Kaempffert, "Science News in Review: Blood and Prejudice: Segregation of White and Negro Donations Brings a Protest," *New York Times,* June 14, 1942.

39. St. John Waddell, "New Currency in the Blood Bank," *Commercial Appeal,* March 9, 1941.

40. L. W. Diggs and Jeannette Spann, "Blood and Plasma Bank at John Gaston Hospital," *Hospitals* July (1942): 10.

41. Diggs, "Clinical Pathology," 239–64.

42. Lemuel W. Diggs Collection, photographs from early blood bank, folder 001-14.

43. *History of the City of Memphis Hospitals Blood Bank* (Memphis, n.d.).

44. Chinn, *Technology and the Logic of American Racism,* 233.

45. John Carruth, "Blood Bank May Save Your Life," *Commercial Appeal,* June 4, 1950.

46. Diggs, "Clinical Pathology," 239–64.

47. Diggs and Spann, "Blood and Plasma Bank," 3.

48. Diggs, "Clinical Pathology," 239–64.

49. L. W. Diggs, "Disputed Points Concerning Technical Procedures Used in Transfusions by the Citrate Method," *Memphis Medical Journal* 17 (1942): 3.

50. L. W. Diggs, "Improved Needle and Observation Tube for the Collection of Blood for Transfusion," *American Journal of Clinical Pathology* 12, no. 11 (1942): 91–92; L. W. Diggs, "The Efficiency of Various Types of Equipment Used in the Collection of Blood for Transfusion," *American Journal of Clinical Pathology* 12, no. 10 (1942): 518–22.

51. L. W. Diggs, "The Milk Bottle as a Blood Transfusion Flask," *American Journal of Clinical Pathology* 13, no. 9 (1943): 101–7.

52. Diggs, "Clinical Pathology," 261.

53. L. W. Diggs and H. B. Turner, "A Shaking Device Used in the Collection of Blood for Transfusion," *Journal of Laboratory and Clinical Medicine* 27, no.8 (1941): 1070–71.

54. L. W. Diggs and J. M. Smith, "A Mechanical Shaker for Transfusion Flasks Using a Standard Electric Motor," *American Journal of Clinical Pathology* 13, no.7 (1943): 67–69.

55. Ann Bell, "A Portrait of Dr. L. W. Diggs," *Tennessee Association of Blood Banks News* 3, no. 2 (1977): 6.

56. Ibid., 7.

57. Chinn, *Technology and the Logic of American Racism,* 233.

58. "Memphis Unprepared, Even for a Peacetime Disaster: The John Gaston Hospital Blood Bank Director Reveals Inadequate Blood Plasma Storage Conditions, Pleads for Action Now," *Memphis Press-Scimitar,* February 3, 1942; "Assure Blood Plasma Supply: Red Cross Will Pay Bill if Memphis Has Need," *Memphis Press-Scimitar,* February 14, 1942; "Blood Bank's Aid to Victims: Speedy Assistance to Those Injured by Tornado," *Memphis Press-Scimitar,* March 19, 1942.

59. John Gaston Hospital, *Report of the John Gaston Hospital for June 1937.* This is taken from a copy of an unpublished, typescript manuscript in the hands of the author.

60. Waddell, "New Currency in the Blood Bank."

61. Carruth, "Blood Bank May Save Your Life."

62. "Memphis Unprepared, Even for a Peacetime Disaster."

63. "Blood Bank's Aid to Victims."

64. Hugh Frank Smith, "Memphis Soon Will be Prepared for Any Big Emergency," *Memphis Press-Scimitar,* 1942. Clipping located in: Health Sciences Historical Collections, the University of Tennessee Health Science Center. See folder LWD 001-18.

65. Ibid., 69.

66. "Plans for Enlarging Blood Banks Speeded," *Memphis Press-Scimitar,* 1942. Clipping located in: Health Sciences Historical Collections, the University of Tennessee Health Science Center. See folder LWD 001-18.

67. Ibid.

68. Ibid.

69. Ada Gilkey, "Blood Plasma Knowledge Is Assembled in Library," *Memphis Press-Scimitar,* no date, newspaper clipping found in: L. W. Diggs Collections, University of Tennessee Health Sciences Historical Collections, folder 001-18.

70. Some examples are "The Segregation of Bloods," *Science* 96, no. 2479 (1942): 8; Kaempffert, "Science News in Review: Blood and Prejudice."

71. Diggs, L. W., "Clinical Pathology," in *History of Medicine in Memphis,* edited by Stewart, Marcus J., William Thomas Black and Mildred Hicks, 239–64, (Memphis: Memphis and Shelby County Medical Society, 1971). See pages 261–62 for quotation.

72. L. W. Diggs, "Red Cross Participation in a Community Blood Bank in Memphis for the Mid-South Area," *Memphis Medical Journal* 25 (1950), 1–4.

Chapter 4

1. Diggs, Notebook, 1924. The notebooks can be found in the Lemuel W. Diggs Collection, University of Tennessee Health Sciences Historical Collections, Memphis. See title page for quotation.

1. Walter Diggs, interview by Richard Nollan, June 13, 2008, audio file. For a broader history, see Laurie B. Green, *Battling the Plantation Mentality: Memphis and the Black Freedom Struggle* (Chapel Hill: University of North Carolina Press, 2007).

2. Hamner, *University of Tennessee, Memphis 75th Anniversary,* 113.

3. Lemuel W. Diggs Collection, folder 001-17-14.

4. R. F. Gillum, "One Blood, Two Biographies," *The Pharos of Alpha Omega Alpha-Honor Medical Society* 61, no. 4 (Fall 1998): 27–28; Spencie Love, *One Blood: The Death and Resurrection of Charles R. Drew* (Chapel Hill: University of North Carolina Press, 1996), 373.

5. The Markle Foundation, begun in 1927 and known for its support of the diffusion of knowledge, funded medical research during and after World War II. See "Markle | History," www.markle.org/our-story/history.

6. For a brief history of the organization, see "Markle | History."

7. Diggs letter to Henry E. Meloney, July 6, 1943, Lemuel W. Diggs Collection, folder 002-6-9.

8. Ibid., 1.

9. Ibid.

10. Ibid., 2.

11. Blackwater is a serious and often fatal complication of chronic malaria.

12. Diggs letter to Henry E. Meloney, July 6, 1943, 2.

13. Ibid.

14. Ibid., 3.

15. Ibid.

16. Walter Diggs, interview by Richard Nollan, June 13, 2008, audio file. Diggs, "Health Care/Human Rights," audio file, Lemuel W. Diggs Collection.

17. L. W. Diggs, "Unitarian Philosophy and Research Philosophy Similar," statement sent to the author by Walter Diggs of his father's Unitarian and scientific beliefs.

18. Ibid.

19. Ibid.

20. Ibid.

21. Diggs, "Health Care/Human Rights."

22. L. W. Diggs, "Letter to Frank C. Jones," p. 1, Manuscript Collection, Lemuel W. Diggs Collection.

23. Ibid.

24. Ibid.

25. Ibid.

26. V. R. Kotlarz, "Tracing Our Roots: Origins of Clinical Laboratory Science," *Clinical Laboratory Science: Journal of the American Society for Medical Technology* 11, no. 1 (January–February 1998): 5–7; V. R. Kotlarz, "Tracing our Roots: The First Clinical Laboratory Scientist," *Clinical Laboratory Science: Journal of the American Society for Medical Technology* 11, no. 2 (March–April 1998): 97–100.

27. Peter Guralnick, Sweet Soul Music: Rhythm and Blues in the Southern Dream of Freedom (Boston: Little, Brown, 1999), 280.

28. Lemuel W. Diggs Collection, in folder LWD 001-07-14.

29. Ibid.

30. Ibid.

31. Ibid.

32. Letter from Diggs to Ann Bell, July 11, 1944, Lemuel W. Diggs Collection.

33. L. W. Diggs, *Transfusion Equipment,* 2,435,820 ed. (U.S. Patent Office, 1948), 1–4.

34. Walter Diggs, interview by Richard Nollan, June 13, 2008, audio file.

35. Diggs letter to Ann Bell, January 4, 1945, Lemuel W. Diggs Collection.

36. John D. Clough, *To Act as a Unit: The Story of the Cleveland Clinic,* 4d ed. (Cleveland: Cleveland Clinic Press, 2004), 270.

37. Diggs letter to Ann Bell, January 4, 1945.

38. Large bone marrow cells with large or multiple nuclei from which platelets are derived.

39. Diggs's Personal notes in Lemuel Diggs Collection. See page two of document number LWD 001-07-14 for quotation.

40. Ibid.

41. Diggs letter to Ann Bell, January 4, 1945, p. 1.

42. Ibid.

43. Diggs letter to Ann Bell, February 9, 1945, Lemuel W. Diggs Collection.

44. Diggs letter to Ann Bell, March 23, 1945, Lemuel W. Diggs Collection.

45. Cecile Heidler letter to Ann Bell, June 28, 1945, Lemuel W. Diggs Collection.

46. Diggs letter to Ann Bell, January 16, 1946, Lemuel W. Diggs Collection.

47. Ibid.

48. Diggs letter to Ann Bell, March 15, 1946, Lemuel W. Diggs Collection.

49. Richard Nollan, interview with Alice Sullivan Diggs, 2011.

50. Diggs letter to Ann Bell, January 16, 1946.

51. Diggs letter to Ann Bell, August 15, 1947, Lemuel W. Diggs Collection.

52. Ibid. Also see personal notes in Lemuel W. Diggs Collection, folder 001-07-14.

53. Walter Diggs, interview by Richard Nollan, Memphis, 2011, audiofile. See also the unpublished manuscript in: Lemuel W. Diggs Collection, University of Tennessee Health Science Center, folder 001-07-14, for quotation.

54. Diggs, Unpublished manuscript, Diggs Collection, folder 001-07-14.

55. Roland H. Alden, *As I Recall: Recollections of Dr. Roland H. Alden, University of Tennessee* (n.p., 1992), 9.

56. Ibid., 12.

57. Dowdy and Crump, *Mayor Crump Don't Like It,* 159; Green, *Battling the Plantation Mentality.*

58. D'Army Bailey and Roger R. Easson, *The Education of a Black Radical: A Southern Civil Rights Activist's Journey, 1959–1964* (Baton Rouge: Louisiana State University Press, 2009), 237.

59. Patricia Adams Graves, conversation with the author, May 2011.

60. Walter Diggs, "Dr. L. W. Diggs and Civil Rights," Memoir, 1–4, unpublished manuscript in: Lemuel W. Diggs Collection, University of Tennessee Health Science Center, folder 005-11.

61. Mabry and Diggs, *History of Medicine in Memphis,* 10.

62. Institute of Medicine, *Medical Education and Societal Needs: A Planning Report for the Health Professions* (Washington, DC: National Academy Press, 1983), 116; Thomas Hale Ham, "Medical Education at Western Reserve University: A Progress Report for the Sixteen Years 1946–1962," *New England Journal of Medicine* 267, no. 18 (1962): 916–23.

63. Starr, *Social Transformation of American Medicine,* esp. "Socialized Medicine and the Cold War," 280–89; Alan Derickson, "The House of Falk: The Paranoid Style in American Health Politics," *American Journal of Public Health* 87, no. 11 (1997): 1836–43.

64. Diggs, "Health Care and Human Rights."

65. Herrick, "Peculiar Elongated and Sickle-Shaped Red Blood Corpuscles," 519.

66. Savitt, "The Invisible Malady," 739–46.

67. Walter Diggs, interview by Richard Nollan, 2011.

Chapter 5

Epigraph: Diggs, Notebook, 1924. The notebooks can be found in the Lemuel W. Diggs Collection, University of Tennessee Health Sciences Historical Collections,

Memphis. This saying is probably taken from Diggs's father. See page 6 for quotation.

1. Diggs letter to Ann Bell, September 4, 1947, Lemuel W. Diggs Collection.

2. L. W. Diggs, "Negative Results in the Treatment of Sickle-Cell Anemia," *American Journal of the Medical Sciences* 187 (1934): 527.

3. Frankie L. Winchester, "The Path from Obscurity: Efforts to Gain Recognition for Sickle Cell Disease, Memphis, 1929–1975," MA thesis, Memphis State University, 1991, 41.

4. L. Pauling and H. A. Itano, "Sickle Cell Anemia a Molecular Disease," *Science* 110, no. 2865 (November 25, 1949): 543–48; also see M. Gormley, "The First 'Molecular Disease': A Story of Linus Pauling, the Intellectual Patron," *Endeavour* 31, no. 2 (Jun 2007): 71–77, and James V. Neel, "The Inheritance of Sickle Cell Anemia." *Science* 110, no. 2846 (1949): 64–66.

5. Diggs, Pulliam, and King, "Bone Changes in Sickle Cell Anemia," 249–60; Winsor and Burch, "Sickle Cell Anemia," 793–96.

6. Richard Nollan, interview with Alice Diggs Sullivan, 2011.

7. Ibid.; "Medical Illustrations of Dorothy Sturm," Memphis, April 29, 2010, University of Tennessee Health Sciences Library, library.uthsc.edu/history/dorothysturmexhibit/.

8. Walter Diggs, conversation with Richard Nollan, May 2008.

9. L. W. Diggs, Dorothy Sturm, and Ann Bell, *The Morphology of Blood Cells,* (Chicago: Abbott Laboratories, 1954). Later editions were titled *The Morphology of Human Blood Cells.*

10. H. D. Chope, "Public Health and Public Medical Care," *California Medicine* 85, no. 4 (Oct 1956): 220–25; "Wagner-Murray-Dingell Bill," *Journal of the American Medical Association* 130 (Apr 27 1946): 1234; "Wagner-Murray-Dingell Social Security or 'Cradle to Grave' Bill (S. 1161; H.R. 2861): Its Place in Relation to Medical Practice," *California and Western Medicine* 59, no. 2 (Aug 1943): 109–11. For a broader discussion, see Starr, *Social Transformation of American Medicine,* 280–86.

11. Walter Diggs interviewed by Richard Nollan, June 13, 2008, audiofile. The author used the Freedom of Information Act and was told that there were no files on Dr. Diggs: David M. Hardy, letter to the author, August, 26, 2010.

12. Lemuel W. Diggs Collection, folder 002-6-17.

13. Diggs, "Health Care and Human Rights."

14. Diggs, "Normal and Abnormal Morphologic Hematology," New Mexico Medical Technologists presentation, no date (probably 1970), audio recording, Lemuel W. Diggs Collection.

15. Lemuel W. Diggs Collection, document 002-6-15.

16. Ibid.

17. Ibid., folder 002-06-20.

18. Alys Lipscomb, "Presented by Dr. Alys Lipscomb at the Presentation of Dr. Diggs' Portrait on May 28, 1961," typescript, p. 1, Lemuel W. Diggs Collection, folder 002-06-49.

19. Kraus, "A Reminiscent Journey," 8.

20. Lipscomb, "Presented by Dr. Alys Lipscomb at the Presentation of Dr. Diggs' Portrait on May 28, 1961," p. 1.

21. Ibid.

22. Ibid.

23. Hamner, *University of Tennessee, Memphis 75th Anniversary*, 75.

24. G. Wayne Dowdy, *Crusades for Freedom: Memphis and the Political Transformation of the American South* (Jackson: University Press of Mississippi, 2010), 183, 41–41, 45–46.

25. O. W. Hyman letter to Sol R. Rubin, March 25, 1955, p. 1, James N. Etteldorf Collection, Manuscript Collection, University of Tennessee Health Sciences Historical Collections, folder 007-12-101.

26. Ibid.

27. Simone, "St. Jude 1962–71: The Formative Years," (presentation, St. Jude Danny Thomas Lecture Series, Memphis, TN, December 16, 2005.

28. J. V. Simone, "A History of St Jude Children's Research Hospital," *British Journal of Haematology* 120, no. 4 (February 2003): 549. Dr. Simone was director of St. Jude from 1983 to 1992.

29. Hazel Fath, *A Dream Come True: The Story of St. Jude Children's Research Hospital and ALSAC* (Dallas: Taylor Publishing Co., 1983), 19.

30. Walter Diggs, "Dr. L. W. Diggs and Civil Rights," 1–4; Diggs letter to H. F. Tamer, May 13, 1961, Lemuel W. Diggs Collection, folder 005-11.

31. Diggs letter to H. F. Tamer, May 13, 1961.

32. Fath, *A Dream Come True*; Danny Thomas, "Congratulations to Diggs for Civitan Award," n.d., recording, Lemuel W. Diggs Collection.

33. "Danny's Dream," www.stjude.org/stjude/v/index.jsp?vgnextoid=d7e8fa3186e70110VgnVCM1000001e0215acRCRD&vgnextchannel=bc67efge870180 10VgnVCM1000000e2015acRCRD; Fath, *A Dream Come True*.

34. Diggs, presentation to second annual meeting of ALSAC, October 4, 1959, Lemuel W. Diggs Collection, folder 002-6-27.

35. Ibid., p. 12.

36. James N. Etteldorf Collection, box 7, folders 1 and 2.

37. Donald Pinkel letter to James Hughes, April 14, 1969, James N. Etteldorf Collection, folder 007-1-88, p. 2.

38. See Etteldorf's marginal notes in letter from James Hughes to Homer Marsh, April 18, 1969, James N. Etteldorf Collection, folder 007-01-74.

39. Lemuel W. Diggs Collection. [AU: Need more specific citation]

40. "Grant Renewed to Trace Strange Malady's Secret: Herff Foundation Again Will Help U-T Seek Facts of Sickle Cell Anemia," *Commercial Appeal*, May 22, 1954, *Commercial Appeal* Morgue File, University of Memphis Library Special Collections, file 80145.

41. L. W. Diggs, "The History of the Sickle Cell Anemia Program and Research in Memphis, Tennessee, 1929–1980," May 1980, p. 2, unpublished manuscript, Lemuel W. Diggs Collection. This manuscript was found in a bound volume in the Diggs Collection marked "Miscellaneous Publications."

42. Ibid.

43. Walter Diggs, interview by Richard Nollan, June 13, 2008).

44. Diggs, Sickle Cell Notebook A, Lemuel W. Diggs Collection, p. 7.

45. Walter Diggs, "Dr. L. W. Diggs and Civil Rights," 1–4. For more on Boyle, see Dowdy and Crump, *Mayor Crump Don't Like It*; Dowdy, *Crusades for Freedom*, 183.

46. "Roosevelt Jamison, 1936–2013," www.peterguralnick.com/post/47106712366/roosevelt-jamison-1936-2013.

47. Peter Guralnick, *Sweet Soul Music: Rhythm and Blues and the Southern Dream of Freedom* (Boston: Little, Brown, 1999), 280.

48. *Memphis Press-Scimitar* Morgue File, series 80145, University of Memphis Library Special Collections.

49. L. W. Diggs, "The Sickle Cell Program in Memphis," in *Unpublished Writings* (Memphis: private, 1977), 3.

50. Kraus, Kraus, and Johnson, "Oral Interview with Alfred P. and Lorraine Kraus," 1.

51. L. M. Kraus, "Formation of Different Haemoglobins in Tissue Culture of Human Bone Marrow Treated with Human Deoxyribonucleic Acid," *Nature* 192 (December 16, 1961): 1055–57.

52. "Cuban Doctor Doesn't Regret Freedom 'Fib'," *Commercial Appeal,* December 9, 1962.

53. "More Funds Needed for Research in Sickle Cell Says Dr. Diggs," *Tri-State Defender,* June 13, 1964 p. 1. This article can be found in Diggs, Sickle Cell Notebook A.

54. "Univ. of Tennessee: Dr. L. W. Diggs, Dept. of Hematology," *ALSAC News* (December 10, 1963); see also Richard Nollan, "Interview with Marion Dugdale, M.D.," Oral Interview, p. 1, University of Tennessee Oral History Program, University of Tennessee Health Science Center, Memphis.

55. "Negroes Raise Funds: Sickle Cell Anemia Research to Be Furthered at UT," *Commercial Appeal,* June 8, 1963); "$3700 More Is Needed to Reach Goal of First Sickle Cell Drive," 1963, clipping found in "Sickle Cell Notebook A" in: L. W. Diggs Collection, Historical Collections, University of Tennessee Health Science Center.

56. "Negroes Help Keep Memphis Anemia Center Open," *Jet* 30, no. 5 (May 5, 1966): 29.

57. "'Sickle Cell' Fight Encourages Unit," *Commercial Appeal,* September 4, 1967, in Diggs, Sickle Cell Notebook A.

58. "Blood Disease Is Keeping Many Negroes on Ground," *Commercial Appeal,* June 4, 1965 in Diggs, Sickle Cell Notebook A.

59. L. W. Diggs, "The Sickle Cell Trait in Relation to the Training and Assignment of Duties in the Armed Forces: I. Policies, Observations, and Studies," *Aviation, Space, and Environmental Medicine* 55, no. 3 (March 1984): 180–85; L. W. Diggs, "The Sickle Cell Trait in Relation to the Training and Assignment of Duties in the Armed Forces: II. Aseptic Splenic Necrosis," *Aviation, Space, and Environmental Medicine* 55, no. 4 (April 1984): 271–76; L. W. Diggs, "The Sickle Cell Trait in Relation to the Training and Assignment of Duties in the Armed Forces: III. Hyposthenuria, Hematuria, Sudden Death, Rhabdomyolysis, and Acute Tubular Necrosis," *Aviation, Space, and Environmental Medicine* 55, no. 5 (May 1984): 358–64; L. W. Diggs, "The Sickle Cell Trait in Relation to the Training and Assignment of Duties in the Armed Forces: IV. Considerations and Recommendations," *Aviation, Space, and Environmental Medicine* 55, no. 6 (Jun 1984): 487–92.

60. "Sickle Cell Center Added to U.T." *University Center-Grams* 18 (February 1965): 1.

61. "Humanitarian Award—Aid to Sickle Cell Anemia, Inc.," photograph, Lemuel W. Diggs Collection, folder 001-03.

62. Hal D. Steward, "Strange Disease Strikes Negroes: Sickle Cell Anemia Said to Affect Significant Part of Population." See Diggs, Sickle Cell Notebook A.

63. Cliff Smith, "Strange Sickle Cell Anemia 'Neglected': 14-Year Life Span," *San Diego Union,* March 26, 1968, in Diggs, Sickle Cell Notebook A, p. 56.

64. L. M. Kraus et al., "Characterization of alpha23GluNH2 in Hemoglobin Memphis: Hemoglobin Memphis/S, a New Variant of Molecular Disease," *Biochemistry* 5, no. 11 (November 1966): 3701–8.

65. Diggs, "Clinical Pathology," 252.

66. Kraus et al., "Characterization of alpha23GluNH2 in Hemoglobin Memphis."; A. P. Kraus et al., "Hemoglobin Memphis/S. A New Variant of Sickle Cell Anemia," *Transactions of the Association of American Physicians* 80 (1967): 297–304; Diggs, "Clinical Pathology," 239–64; Alfred Kraus, Lorraine Kraus, Interview by James Gibb Johnson, March 19, 2003, in: University of Tennessee Health Sciences Historical Collections, Oral History Collection. 1, Diggs, "Clinical Pathology," 252.

67. L. M. Kraus and A. P. Kraus, "Carbamoyl Phosphate Mediated Inhibition of the Sickling of Erythrocytes in Vitro," *Biochemical and Biophysical Research Communications* 44, no. 6 (September 17, 1971): 1381–87; L. M. Kraus and A. P. Kraus, "Carbamoyl Phosphate Mediated Inhibition of the Sickling of Erythrocytes in Whole Blood in Vitro from Sickle Cell Anemia Patients," *Journal of Laboratory and Clinical Medicine* 78, no. 5 (November 1971): 843–44.

68. "Quick Test for Sickle Hemoglobin," JAMA 206 (November 11, 1968), 1438; "New Procedure for Detection of Sickle Hemoglobin," *Memphis and Mid-South Medical Journal* 44 (January, 1969), 20. See also D. M. Canning and R. G. Huntsman, "An Assessment of Sickledex as an Alternative to the Sickling Test," *Journal of Clinical Pathology* 23 (1970): 736–37; M. Susan Ballard et al., "A New Diagnostic Test for Hemoglobin S," *Journal of Pediatrics* 76, no. 1 (1970): 117–19; R. G. Huntsman et al., "A Rapid Whole Blood Solubility Test to Differentiate the Sickle-Cell Trait from Sickle-Cell Anaemia," *Journal of Clinical Pathology* 23, no. 9 (1970): 781–83.

69. L. W. Diggs and D. L. Williams, "Treatment of Painful Sickle Cell Crises with Papaverine: Preliminary Report," *Southern Medical Journal* 56 (May 1963): 472–74.

70. L. Barreras and L. W. Diggs, "Bicarbonates, Ph and Percentage of Sickled Cells in Venous Blood of Patients in Sickle Cell Crisis," *American Journal of the Medical Sciences* 247 (June 1964): 710–18.

71. Frankie L. Winchester, Alfred P. Kraus, and Memphis State University, *Sickle Cell Anemia Research in Memphis: Interview with Alfred P. Kraus, M.D., October 27, 1989* (Memphis: Oral History Research Office, Memphis State University, 1989).

72. L. W. Diggs, "Background Information and Opinions Concerning the Sickle Cell Program in Memphis," 1974, 3, Unpublished Writings, Lemuel W. Diggs Collection.

73. Dowdy, *Crusades for Freedom,* 183, 62.

74. Walter Diggs, "Dr. L. W. Diggs and Civil Rights," 1–4.

75. Gene H. Stollerman, *Medicine, A Love Story: The 20th Century Odyssey of an American Professor of Medicine* (Parker, CO: Outskirts Press, Inc., 2012).

76. Robert B. Baker et al., "African American Physicians and Organized Medicine, 1846–1968: Origins of a Racial Divide," *JAMA: Journal of the American Medical Association* 300, no. 3 (2008): 306–14.

77. Lemuel W. Diggs Collection, folder 002-6-16. See also W. Michael Byrd and Linda A. Clayton, "An American Health Dilemma: A History of Blacks in the Health System," *Journal of the National Medical Association* 84, no. 2 (1992): 189–200.

78. L. W. Diggs, "Why Negroes Should Be Admitted as Regular Members," 1956. Unpublished manuscript in: Lemuel W. Diggs Collection, Health Sciences Historical Collections, University of Tennessee. See folder LWD 002-06-16.

79. Ibid.

80. Ibid.

81. Charles M. Payne, *I've Got the Light of Freedom: The Organizing Tradition and the Mississippi Freedom Struggle* (Berkeley: University of California Press, 1995), 34–35; Michael W. Fuquay, "Civil Rights and the Private School Movement in Mississippi, 1964–1971," *History of Education Quarterly* 42, no. 2 (July 1, 2002): 159–80.

82. Scott Ware, "Cell Life Gives Wing to Spirit," *Commercial Appeal,* December 2, 1975, in Diggs, Sickle Cell Center Notebook B.

83. Ibid.; Robert B. Patterson letter to Diggs, September 26, 1957, folder 002-6-23, Lemuel W. Diggs Collection.

84. Patterson letter to Diggs, September 26, 1957.

85. Ibid.

86. Ibid.

87. Ibid., p. 2.

88. Ware, "Cell Life Gives Wing to Spirit."

89. Walter Diggs, "Dr. L. W. Diggs and Civil Rights," 1–4.

90. "Nation: The Assassination," *Time,* April 12, 1968.

91. Ibid.

92. Ibid.

93. Albert Biggs, Interview by Bill Robinson, (Memphis: University of Tennessee, February 19, 1998), 1–20; Maston Callison, Interview by Robert Summit, (Memphis: University of Tennessee Health Science Center, 1997), 1–14. At the time of the strike, Dr. Biggs was a urologist at the University of Tennessee and Dr. Callison was dean of the College of Medicine.

94. Walter Diggs, "Dr. L. W. Diggs and Civil Rights," 1–4.

95. Lemuel W. Diggs Collection, folder 005-11.

96. Ibid.

97. Ibid.

98. Smith, "Strange Sickle Cell Anemia 'Neglected.'"

99. Ibid.

100. Ibid.

Chapter 6

Epigraph: Diggs, Notebook, 1924. The notebooks can be found in the Lemuel W. Diggs Collection, University of Tennessee Health Sciences Historical Collections, Memphis. This saying is probably taken from Diggs's father. See page 90 for quotation.

1. "Special Message to the Congress Proposing a National Health Strategy," February 18, 1971, www.presidency.ucsb.edu/ws/index.php?pid=3311#axzz1m6DoQ2nC.

2. William Hines, "Sickle-Cell Anemia: 'Stylish' Disease," *Commercial Appeal,* November 28, 1971. Additional details on the Black Panthers and sickle cell screening can be found in Alondra Nelson, *Body and Soul: The Black Panther Party and the Fight Against Medical Discrimination* (Minneapolis: University of Minnesota Press, 2013).

3. Winchester, Kraus, and Memphis State University, *Sickle Cell Anemia Research in Memphis,* 26–27; Wailoo, *Dying in the City of the Blues,* 338, 193.

4. Hines, "Sickle-Cell Anemia."

5. Ibid.; Nicole S. Lewis, "Sickle Cell Threat," *Commercial Appeal,* December 22, 1971; "Congress Against Sickle Cell," *Nature* 233 (1971): 517–18.

6. Charles Thornton, "Science Unlocking Sickle Cell," *Commercial Appeal,* January 11, 1972, 13.

7. Diggs, "Background Information and Opinions Concerning the Sickle Cell Program in Memphis," 1.

8. Ibid.; Thornton, "Science Unlocking Sickle Cell," 13.

9. Diggs, "Background Information and Opinions Concerning the Sickle Cell Program in Memphis," 16, 6.

10. Walter Diggs, interview by Richard Nollan, (Memphis: September 16, 2011).

11. Ibid., 3.

12. Wailoo, *Dying in the City of the Blues,* 186–87; Mary L. Hampton et al., "Sickle Cell 'Nondisease': A Potentially Serious Public Health Problem," *American Journal of Diseases of Children* 128, no. 1 (1974): 58–61.

13. Diggs, "Background Information and Opinions Concerning the Sickle Cell Program in Memphis," 3.

14. Ibid.

15. Ibid.

16. "Busing Creates Sickle Problem," newspaper clipping in: Sickle Cell Notebook B, Historical Collections, University of Tennessee Health Science Center. See page 65 for clipping. in Diggs, Sickle Cell Center Notebook B.

17. Diggs, "Background Information and Opinions Concerning the Sickle Cell Program in Memphis," 16, 3.

18. Ibid.

19. Ibid. A. P. Kraus, *The University of Tennessee Center for the Health Sciences, Memphis, Tennessee: Comprehensive Center for Research and Service in Sickle Cell Disease* (Memphis: University of Tennessee Center for the Health Sciences), 1, brochure, in Diggs, Sickle Cell Center Notebook B. Also see L. W. Diggs and Ernestine Flowers, "High School Athletes with the Sickle Cell Trait (Hb A/S)," *Journal of the National Medical Association* 68, no. 6 (1976): 492–97; Diggs and Flowers, *The Socio-Economic Problems in Sickle Cell Anemia.*

20. Diggs and Flowers, *The Socio-Economic Problems in Sickle Cell Anemia,* 9; L. W. Diggs and E. Flowers, "Sickle Cell Anemia in the Home Environment: Observations on the Natural History of the Disease in Tennessee Children," *Clinical Pediatrics* 10, no. 12 (1971): 697–700.

21. Hampton et al., "Sickle Cell 'Nondisease,'" 58–61; also see Nelson, *Body and Soul.*

22. Hampton et al., "Sickle Cell 'Nondisease,'" 58.

23. Melinda Gormley, "It's in the Blood: The Varieties of Linus Pauling's Work on Hemoglobin and Sickle Cell Anemia," PhD diss., University of Oregon, 2007, 126; "Mastering Genetics: Pauling and Eugenics," http://paulingblog. wordpress.com/2009/02/24/mastering-genetics-pauling-and-eugenics/ (accessed August 31, 2013).

24. William Cole, "Dr. Jackson's War on Sickle Cell," *The Smithsonian* (June 1972): 67–70.

25. L. W. Diggs, "Genetic Counseling for Sickle-Cell-Disease Carriers," *New England Journal of Medicine* 285, no. 22 (November 1971): 1266.

26. Diggs, letter to Loretta Jo Shaw, May 19, 1973, p. 1, Lemuel W. Diggs Collection, folder 002-08.

27. A thorough history of genetic counseling in the twentieth century can be found in Alexandra Minna Stern, *Telling Genes: The Story of Genetic Counseling in America* (Baltimore: Johns Hopkins University Press, 2012); see also M. Gormley, "Scientific Discrimination and the Activist Scientist: L.C. Dunn and the Professionalization of Genetics and Human Genetics in the United States," *Journal of the History of Biology* 42, no. 1 (Spring 2009): 33–72.

28. Diggs, letter to Shaw, May 19,1973. See page 2 for quotation.

29. Diggs, "Genetic Counseling for Sickle-Cell-Disease Carriers."

30. Diggs, letter to Shaw, May 19, 1973. See page 2 for quotation.

31. Ibid., 1266–67.

32. Ibid.

33. Ibid. See Diggs letter to Wilde Rinehart, October 19, 1978, Lemuel W. Diggs Collection, folder 002-9-13.

34. Diggs letter to Wilde Rinehart, October 19, 1978, Lemuel W. Diggs Collection, folder 002-9-13.

35. Danny Thomas letter to Diggs, January 15, 1975, Lemuel W. Diggs Collection, folder 002-8-27.

36. Walter Diggs, "Dr. L. W. Diggs and Civil Rights," 1–4; Edward Soma, Richard Shadyac, and Danny Thomas letter to Diggs, January 13, 1976, Lemuel W. Diggs Collection, folder 002-8-24.

37. Diggs letter to Colin Vor der Bruegge, August 16, 1976, Lemuel W. Diggs Collection, folder 002-8-53.

38. Peter Alan Harper, "Sickle Cell Pioneer, Group Cited," *Commercial Appeal,* April 27, 1981. Clipping found in File Card Index, *The Press Scimitar* Morgue File, University of Memphis, Ned McWherter Library, Special Collections, file 80145.

39. Ibid. See various letters in box 2, folder 09 of the L. W. Diggs Collection.

40. *Commercial Appeal,* August 29, 1985, in Lemuel W. Diggs Collection, folder 002-10.

41. Diggs letter to Albert Joseph, July 9, 1985, Manuscript Collection, James N. Etteldorf Collection, folder 002-19.

42. Diggs, letter to Charles H. Hennekens, December 8, 1988, Lemuel W. Diggs Collection, folder 002-10-42; Diggs letter to Graham Serjeant, August 10, 1989, Lemuel W. Diggs Collection, folder 002-10-43.

43. Diggs, letter to Hennekens, 1988.

44. For example, see Diggs letter to Peggy D. Friend, January 26, 1987, Lemuel W. Diggs Collection, folder LWD 002-10-28.

45. Hugh Scott letter to Diggs, December 4, 1986, Lemuel W. Diggs Collection, folder 002-10-34.

46. Diggs letter to Titus H. J. Huisman, January 3, 1981, Lemuel W. Diggs Collection, folder 002-9-35.

47. Ibid.

48. Ibid.

49. "Civitan: About Us," http://www.civitan.com/template.php?id=117.

50. Thomas, "Congratulations to Diggs."

51. Diggs letter to Ann Bell, November 24, 1991, Lemuel W. Diggs Collection, folder 002-10-64.

52. Diggs, Sturm, and Bell, *The Morphology of Human Blood Cells,* 5th ed. (Abbott Park, IL: Abbott Laboratories, 1985), 89.

53. Ann Bell letter to Beatrice Diggs, December 30, 1993, Lemuel W. Diggs Collection, folder 002-10-69.

54. Bell letter to Diggs, January 4, 1992, p. 2, Lemuel W. Diggs Collection, folder 002-11-1.

55. Ibid., p. 3.

56. L. W. Diggs, letter to Hillary Rodham Clinton, April 2, 1993, in: L. W. Diggs Collection, folder 002-11-24; L. W. Diggs, "Recommendation to the Task Force on National Health Care Reform," typescript manuscript, April 7, 1993 in: Lemuel W. Diggs Collection, folder 002-11-25.

57. Carol H. Rasco letter to Diggs, August 16, 1993, Lemuel W. Diggs Collection, folder 002-11-34.

58. L. W. Diggs, "Sickle Cell Hemoglobinopathies: The Need for Postmortem Examinations," manuscript completed posthumously by Ann Bell with the help of colleagues, though not published, in: L. W. Diggs Collection, folders 003-14 and 003-15.

59. Richard Nollan, interview with Alice Diggs Sullivan, 2011.

60. James Kingsley, "Dr. Diggs Dies at 95; Sickle Cell, St. Jude Work Serve as Legacies," *Commercial Appeal,* January 10, 1995, B1.

61. Gabrielle C. L. Songe, "Tribute to Dr. L. W. Diggs: A Legendary Figure Who Made an Outstanding Contribution in the Field of Sickle Cell Disease," *Tri-State Defender,* 1995, 5A, clipping found in the L. W. Diggs Collection, folder 004-22.

62. Lecture notes, Lemuel W. Diggs Collection, folder 004-22.

63. Ann Bell, "Memorial Service—January 15, 1995: Talk by Ann Bell," autograph manuscript, 1995, Lemuel W. Diggs Collection, folder 004-22.

Conclusion

1. Walter Diggs, interview by Richard Nollan, Memphis, 2011, audio file.

2. Diggs, "Notebook of Collected Sayings," 1924.

3. Walter Diggs, "We Celebrate Beatrice Diggs and Her Full Life," notes given to the author by Walter Diggs, p. 1.

4. Walter Diggs, interview by Richard Nollan, Memphis, June 13, 2008, audio file. Green, *Battling the Plantation Mentality.*

Index

Page numbers in **boldface** refer to illustrations.

laboratory testing (*cont'd*) in, 87–88; growing dependency on, 64–65; for sickle cell, 43; sickle cell detection technology, 130

labor issues, Diggs's commentary on, 134–35

Landsteiner, Karl, 68

Le Bonheur Children's Hospital, 119

Lemuel Whitley Diggs Professorship in Medicine, 148

Lipscomb, Alys, **108**, 117–18

liver extract: Diggs's sickle cell research and use of, 34–35, 37–38; pernicious anemia therapy with, 19–21

Liver Extract, 343; Eli Lily & Co. development of, 21

Ludmerer, Kenneth M., 13–14, 64

Mabry, Thelma W., 52

malaria: Diggs's research on, 83–86, 171n11; thalassemia and, 51

Marcus Welby, M.D. (television show), 138

Markle Foundation, Diggs's Fellowship from, 84, 88

Martin Luther King Medical Achievement Award, Diggs as recipient of, 147

M*A*S*H (television show), 138

Mason, George, 10, 86, 116

Mason, Verne, 44

maternal mortality rates, transfusion technology and reduction of, 69–70

Mayo Clinic, 68

McCann, William, 17–18, 23, 34, 88

McFarland, Patricia LaPointe, 28–29

McGehee, Lucius, 52–53, 69

medical illustration, Diggs's use in research of, 16, 49–50, 114–15

medical literature: absence of sickle cell research in, 40–42; collection of sickle research in, 136–47

Medicare, 141

Meharry University Medical School, 146

Memphis, Tennessee: Diggs's life in, 29–33; environmental health problems in, 27–28; impact of Great Depression on, 32–33; labor strikes in, 134–35; sanitation system in, 28–29; sickle cell disease in, 44–45

Memphis and Shelby County Medical Society, 7–8, 44–45, 120, 132, 154, 156

Memphis City Hospital: Diggs's work with, 2–7, 35–36, 47–48; expansion of, 60–61; history of, 40; Pathology Institute at, 38; pediatric unit in, 119; public health initiatives and, 29–30; sickle disease in, 45

Memphis Commercial Appeal, 33

Memphis Medical Society, 134

Memphis Press-Scimitar newspapers, 79

Memphis Public Affairs Forum, 78

Memphis Regional Sickle Cell Council (MRSCC), 140, 142

Memphis Research Coordinating Committee, 140

Mendelian genetics, sickle cell disease and, 44–45, 165n64

Methodist Church, Diggs's dissatisfaction with, 9–12, 31

Meyer, Jerome, 43

microscope, Diggs's use of, 16, 34

Minot, George Richard, 19

Morehouse College, 146

The Morphology of Blood Cells (Diggs), 115, 150

Moshier, Beatrice. *See* Diggs, Beatrice Moshier

Mount Vernon College, 14

Murphy, William Parry, 19

"My Ambitions" (Diggs), 1

"My Idea of a Man" (Diggs), 1

Nash, Thomas Palmer, 23, 126

national health insurance, Diggs's interest in, 10, 97–98, 115–16

National Institutes of Health: sickle cell research funding from, 7, 127, 138–40

National Library of Medicine, 146

National Medical Association, 132
National Sickle Cell Disease Advisory
    Board, 138
New England Journal of Medicine,
    144
Nixon, Richard M., 137–38, 143
nutritional research, Diggs's
    participation in, 18–20

Olim, Charles, 69
Orthro Diagnostics, 130
OsirUS Club, 128
Osler, William, 13, 34, 41, 154
Outstanding Citizen Award from the
    Civitan Clubs, 149
Overton, Watkins, 29, 78

Packer, Henry, 117
Packer, Lou, 117
Paine, Thomas, 86
papaverine, sickle cell therapy with,
    131
pathology, Diggs's belief in, 6–7, 17–
    18, 22–23, 38–39, 65–66
patient care, Diggs's commitment to,
    65–66
Patterson, Robert B., 133–1334
Pauling, Linus, 113, 143–44
pellagra, early research on, 37–38
pernicious anemia, Diggs's research
    on, 19–21, 34
Petrie, John, 31
physician-scientist model, Diggs's
    embrace of, 33–34
Pinkel, Donald, 122–23
plasma donations, drive for, 84
Poitier, Sidney, 138–39
politics: Diggs's involvement, 97–99,
    135–36, 156; in health research
    funding, 137–38
Practical Nurses Association, 128
public health: blood banks as tool in,
    78–79; impact of Great Depression
    on, 54–57; Memphis initiatives in,
    29–30; racism in, 45–46
Public Health Service Act, 138
Public Works Administration, 60–61

Quick, W. E., 59–60

racism: blood bank segregation of
    blood and, 66–67, 70–81, **102**;
    Diggs's experiences with, 3–6,
    155–56; in medicine, 44–46, 125,
    133–34; postwar challenges to, 95–
    96; sickle cell disease and, 44–45,
    72–73, 124–25, 131–34, 165n64;
    suspicion of medical research and,
    56–57, 124–25, 128–29, 143–46
Randolph-Macon College, Diggs as
    student at, 10–13
religion, Diggs's attitudes about, 9–12,
    30–31, 86–87, 156
Robscheit-Robbins, Frieda, 18–19
Roosevelt, Franklin D., 61, 115
Roosevelt, Teddy, 26
rural medicine, shortage of physicians
    for, 39, 166n97

Sabin, Florence Rena, 15–16
Schering Company, 130
Schmeisser, Harry Christian, 21–23,
    32, 38, 65
Scianni, Joseph L., 49–50, 114
scientific research: African American
    suspicion of, 55–57; on blood-
    group compatibility, 66–81; Diggs's
    belief in, 36–37, 41–43, 86–87,
    163n31; postwar expansion of,
    95–97
Scott, Hugh, 149
segregation: blood bank formation
    and barriers of, 80–81; in blood
    banks, 4–6, 66–67, 70–81, **102**;
    of blood units, 4–6; Diggs's
    experiences with, 3–4, 27–28,
    155–56; integration of Memphis
    institutions and, 131–32; in
    medicine, 37, 44–46, 125, 133–34;
    in Memphis, 29–30, 39–40; postwar
    challenges to, 95–96; sickle cell
    anemia as basis for, 72–73, 131–33;
    at Sickle Cell Center, 140–41
Serjeant, Graham, 151
Sheldon, Doris, 127

shunting techniques, Diggs's interest in, 15

sickle cell anemia: absence of research on, 40–41; cell morphology in, 47–49; collection of literature relating to, 136–47; Diggs's research on, 2–3, 6–7, 14–17, 34–35, 37–38, 41–43, 47–48, 89–90, 94–95, **105–7**, 155; early theories concerning, 43–45; educational programs about, 141–42; federal research funding for, 137–40; hereditary nature of, 44–45; heritability of, 34–45, 47–49, 138, 165n64; pathology of, 50–52; postwar research on, 113–14; racial politics and, 44–45, 72–73, 124–25, 131–34, 165n64; screening tests for, 130, 143–46; Sickle Cell Center founded by Diggs, 111–36; skin ulcers associated with, 3, 40, 43, 45, 49, 99, 130–31, 149; symptoms of, 40–41; therapy research for, 130–31

Sickle Cell Center: community and educational outreach programs at, 140–42; federal funding for, 139–40; founding of, 5, 7, 114–15, 123–36, 155

sickle cell trait, 113, 139, 143–46

Sickledex, 130

Sickle-IS, 130

Sickle Quik, 130

Sickle-Sol, 130

"The Sickle Cell Crisis" (Diggs), 126

Sigma Phi Epsilon, Diggs as member of, 12

Simone, J. V., 120

Smith, E. C., 51

Smith, J. M., 77

social welfare, Diggs on health and, 85–86

Southern Christian Leadership Conference, 147

Southern Medical Association, Diggs's presentation on sickle cell at, 48–51

Spanish-American War (1898), 11

Spanish Civil War, blood banks established during, 66

Spann, Jeanette, 77, 83, **108**

"Special Message to the Congress Proposing a National Health Strategy," 137

spleen, sickle cell disease and enlargement of, 50–53

splenectomy, sickle cell disease and role of, 52–53

Stargel, Willie, 138

Steinberg, B., 48

St. Jude Children's Research Hospital: establishment of, 5, 8, **105**, 114, 118–36, 139, 149; National Advisory Board of, 146; proposed relocation of, 147–48

St. Jude Steering Committee, 120

Stollerman, Gene, 131–32

Stritch, Samuel Cardinal, 118

Strong Memorial Hospital (Rochester, New York), 17–18, 34, 123

Student Army Training Corps, Diggs's participation in, 10

Sturm, Dorothy, 16, 114–15, 150

Sydenstricker, Virgil P., 44, 48

Tate, Maurice, 127

Tauber, Alfred J., 44

technological innovation: blood bank expansion and, 74–81; Diggs's advocacy for, 87–88; transfusion research and, 68–70

Temple Men's Club, 70

Tetralogy of Fallot, 15

thalassemia, early research on, 18, 34, 37

Thomas, Danny, 8, **105**, 114, 118–21, 127, 146, 149

Thomas, Vivien, 37

Tobey, Frank T., 118–19

transfusion research: cross-matching techniques, 77–78; Diggs's involvement in, 65–81; Diggs's patent for transfusion device and, 89–90; increase in transfusion procedures and, 78–81; racial segregation and, 66–67, 70–81; technological innovation in, 68–70. *See also* blood banks

Tri-State Defender newspaper, 128, 151

tropical disease, Diggs's research on, 6, 84–85

Truman, Harry S., 115, 131

Tuskegee Syphilis Project, 7, 141, 166n99

Unitarian Universalist Church, 18, 30–31, 86

University of Nashville Medical College (UNMC), 26

University of Rochester: Diggs on faculty of, 88–89; Diggs's internship and residency at, 2, 16–20, 34, **101**

University of Tennessee Medical Units: Depression-era economics and, 61–64; Diggs's career with, 2–3, 6–7, 21–23, 25–57, 89–90; establishment of, 25–26; expansion of, 60–61; sickle cell research at, 47–48, 94–95; St. Jude Children's Hospital and, 122–23; World War II and expansion of, 83–84, 87–88, 95–97

Upshaw, Jeff, 127

U.S. Public Health Service, 115, 127, 141

Vanderbilt University, 37, 124–25

Virginia Constitution, 86

Virginia Declaration of Rights, 10, 86, 116

Virginian of the Year Award, Diggs as recipient of, 147

Virginia Press Association, 147

Volunteers in Aid of Sickle Cell Anemia, Inc., 129

"von Jaksch anemia," 51, 165n80

Vorder Bruegge, Colin F., 77, 94–95

Voting Rights Act of 1965, 141

Wagner-Murray-Dingell Bill, 97–99, 115–16

Wailoo, Keith, 72

Ward Burdick Award, Diggs as recipient of, 129

A Warm December (film), 138–39

West African Medical Journal, 51

Whipple, George, 17–20, 23, 27, 34, 37–38

William F. Bowld Hospital, 128

William R. Moore School of Technology, 77

Wilson, Woodrow, 10

Winn, R. H., 12

Wintrobe, Maxwell, 41

yellow fever epidemics (Memphis, Tennessee), 28

Yellow Jacket (Randolph-Macon yearbook), 10

Young Men's Christian Association, Diggs's involvement with, 11

Zonta Club, 79–80